"十三五" 职业教育

药学专业英语

Pharmaceutical English

张春玉　　黄国辉　　主编

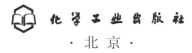

化学工业出版社

·北京·

本教材立足于高职高专学生的学习特点，内容紧扣药学类重点专业课程的重点知识，符合行业的发展，知识点较新，各单元内容比例适当、难易程度适中，英文表达纯正。

全书分为四个单元，共 19 课。第一单元为药学类各专业必备的基本知识，内容主要涉及常见的微生物和人体的结构及疾病等知识；第二单元主要介绍药品生产技术的理论基础；第三单元主要对药品经营与管理进行了介绍；第四单元主要介绍了生物制药方面的相关知识。以上四个单元的内容涵盖了药学类专业的基本知识，各专业可以根据本专业人才培养目标的实际需要对各单元自由组合进行教学。

This textbook is based on the learning characteristics of higher vocational college students. The content is closely related to the key knowledge of the major courses of pharmacy. The content is in line with the development of the industry with the new knowledge. It features appropriate ratio of each unit，moderate difficulty and the pure English expressions.

The book is divided into four units，with a total of 19 lessons. The first unit is the essential area of the pharmaceutical majors that includes microorganism and human body structure as well as disease. The second unit introduces basic theory of production technique for pharmacy. The third unit describes related management and administration for pharmacy. The fourth unit introduces biopharmaceutics. These four units cover the basic knowledge of pharmaceutical major. Therefore，pharmacy professionals can combine units freely and teach according to the actual needs of personnel training purposes.

图书在版编目（CIP）数据

药学专业英语/张春玉，黄国辉主编. —北京：化学
工业出版社，2019.11
"十三五"职业教育规划教材
ISBN 978-7-122-35222-4

Ⅰ.①药… Ⅱ.①张…②黄… Ⅲ.①药物学-英语-
职业教育-教材 Ⅳ.①R9

中国版本图书馆 CIP 数据核字（2019）第 212210 号

责任编辑：迟　蕾　张春娥　　　　　　装帧设计：王晓宇
责任校对：杜杏然

出版发行：化学工业出版社（北京市东城区青年湖南街 13 号　邮政编码 100011）
印　　刷：北京京华铭诚工贸有限公司
装　　订：三河市振勇印装有限公司
710mm×1000mm　1/16　印张 10¼　字数 177 千字
2020 年 1 月北京第 1 版第 1 次印刷

购书咨询：010-64518888　　　　　　售后服务：010-64518899
网　　址：http://www.cip.com.cn
凡购买本书，如有缺损质量问题，本社销售中心负责调换。

定　　价：36.00 元　　　　　　　　　　　　　　　　版权所有　违者必究

前　言

本教材立足于高职高专学生的学习特点，内容紧扣药学类各专业课程的重点知识，符合行业的发展，知识点较新，各单元内容比例适当、难易程度适中，英文表达纯正。

全书共分为四个单元，总共19课。第一单元为药学类各专业必备的基本知识，内容主要涉及常见的微生物和人体的结构及疾病等知识，本单元共计4课（第1课由长春职业技术学院于丽静老师编写，第2课由吉林农业大学郭立泉老师编写，第3课由吉林省人民医院史美龙老师编写，第4课由江苏食品药品职业技术学院周敏老师编写）；第二单元主要介绍药品生产技术的理论基础，本单元共计4课（第5课、6课和7课由江苏食品药品职业技术学院孔庆新老师编写，第8课由长春职业技术学院毛春玲老师编写）；第三单元主要对药品经营与管理进行介绍，共计4课（第9课由长春职业技术学院王然老师编写，第10课和第11课由东北师范大学生命科学学院黄国辉老师编写，第12课由长春职业技术学院刘颖老师编写）；第四单元主要介绍生物制药方面的相关知识，共计7课（第13课由长春职业技术学院刘洋老师编写，第14课由石家庄职业技术学院梁堃老师编写，第15课由石家庄职业技术学院孙百虎老师编写，第16课由长春职业技术学院宋笛老师编写，第17课、18课和19课由长春职业技术学院张春玉老师编写）；另外，李冬寒和张国英老师也参加了部分内容的编写。以上四个单元的知识涵盖了药学类专业的基本知识，各专业可以根据专业人才培养目标的实际需要对各单元自由组合进行教学。本教材由张春玉、黄国辉任主编，孔庆新、郭立泉、刘洋为副主编。

每单元于专题课前都列有学习目标，使学生明确本专题应掌握的重点内容。课文中均有情境导入、知识介绍和应用实例等使学生在掌握知识的同时明确其具体应用。课后部分有课文词汇、重点小结、课后检测、问题讨论及相关的延伸阅读材料，使学生在课后能自主复习检测并有针对性地提高阅读能力。教材的最后附有附录，可以方便学生自主查询相关专业词汇。本书的内容及结构设计充分体现了高职高专的以职业能力培养为主线的教学要求，可以作为高职高专药学类各专业学生专业英语学习的教材和参考书。

本教材的编写凝聚了全体参编人员的努力，教材编写工作量大、任务繁重，尽管我们做了最大努力，但仍可能存在疏漏和不足之处，竭诚希望广大读者批评指正。

编者

2019.7

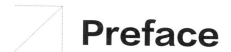

Preface

　　This textbook is based on the learning characteristics of higher vocational college students. The content is closely related to the key knowledge of the major courses of pharmacy. The content is in line with the development of the industry with the new knowledge. It features appropriate ratio of each unit, moderate difficulty and the pure English expressions.

　　The book is divided into four units, with a total of 19 lessons. The first unit is the essential area of the pharmaceutical majors that includes microorganism and human body structure as well as disease. This unit is composed of 4 lessons (The 1st lesson is written by Yu Lijing from Changchun Vocational Institute of Technology. The 2nd lesson is written by Guo Liquan from Jilin Agricultural University. The 3rd lesson is written by Shi Meilong from the Jilin Provincial People's Hospital. The 4th lesson is written by Zhou Min from Jiangsu Food & Pharmaceutical Science College).

　　The second unit introduces basic theory of production technique for pharmacy. This unit consists of 4 lessons (The 5th, the 6th and the 7th lessons are written by Kong Qingxin from Jiangsu Food & Pharmaceutical Science College. The 8th lesson is written by Mao Chunling from Changchun Vocational Institute of Technology).

　　The third unit describes related management and administration for pharmacy. There are 4 lessons in this unit (The 9th lesson is written by Wang Ran from Changchun Vocational Institute of Technology. The 10th and the 11th lessons are written by Huang Guohui from life science, Northeast Normal University. The 12th lesson is written by Liu Ying from Changchun Vocational Institute of Technology).

　　The fourth unit introduces biopharmaceutics. This unit consists of 7 lessons (The 13th lesson is written by Liu Yang from Changchun Vocational Institute of Technology. The 14th lesson is written by Liang Kun from Shijiazhuang Vocational Technology Institute. The 15th lesson is written by Sun Baihu from Shijiazhuang Vocational Technology Institute. The 16th is written by Song Di from Changchun Vocational Institute of Technology. The 17th, 18th and 19th lessons are written by Zhang Chunyu from Changchun Vocational Institute of Technology).

Some of contents are written by Li Donghan and Zhang Guoying.

These four units cover the basic knowledge of pharmaceutical major. Therefore, pharmacy professionals can combine units freely and teach according to the actual needs of personal training purposes.

Zhang Chunyu and Huang Guohui are chief editors. Kong Qingxin, Guo Liquan and Liu Yang are associate editors.

There is a learning goal in each unit before the subject, so students can make clear the key content of the subject. The introduction of situation and the knowledge and application examples enable the students to understand their specific application. Further, the vocabulary, the conclusion of key knowledge, quiz, question discussion and the related expanded reading materials make students independently review and improve their reading ability after class. The appendix can facilitate students' independent inquiry of relevant professional vocabulary. The above content and structure design fully reflect the teaching requirements of vocational ability training in higher vocational colleges. Therefore, this book can be used as a textbook as well as reference for professional English learning in higher vocational colleges.

The book has condensed the efforts of all the participants and we express our sincere respect and gratitude to all of them. The workload of textbooks is heavy and the tasks are arduous. Even though we have tried our best, we still can't avoid shortcomings. We sincerely hope readers will criticize and correct them.

July 2019

Index 目 录

Unit 1　Human Body and Microorganisms
第一单元　人体和微生物

Unit 2　Basic Theory of Production Technique for Pharmacy
第二单元　药品生产技术理论基础

Unit 3　Medicine Sale and Management
第三单元　药品销售和管理

Unit 4　Biopharmaceutics
第四单元　生物制药

Appendix
附　录

Reference
（参考文献）

Unit 1

Human Body and Microorganisms
第一单元　人体和微生物

🖊 Study Objective（学习目标）

1. Grasping the pharmaceutical English terms.
2. Learning how to translate pharmaceutical English.
3. Getting familiar with the important knowledge of human body and microorganisms.

Lesson 1　Microorganisms Around Us
第一课　常见微生物

🖊 Situational Entry（情境导入）

　　Around us，there is an invisible world——the microbial world. Microbes have been existed for thousands of years，and they are everywhere. Even washing every part of our body all of the time，we're still covered with a cloud of microorganisms（microbes）. A few of these are listed below（Fig. 1-1）.

　　Both in vivo and in vitro，there are a large number of microorganisms inhabiting our bodies. Although bacteria are the most important group，there are also single-celled organisms called archaea，as well as fungi，viruses and other mi-

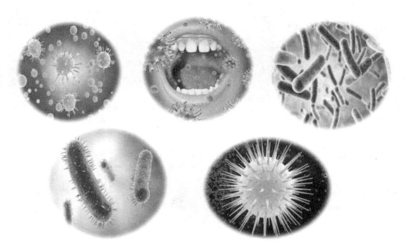

Fig. 1-1   Microbes around us

croorganisms. They are collectively referred to as human microflora. Microorganisms in the human body play many important roles in protecting our immune system and providing nutrition for human cells.

Information about microorganism（microbe）(微生物相关知识)

What is a microbe?（什么是微生物?）

The word microorganism（microbe）is used to describe an organism that is too small to be seen without the use of a microscope. Viruses，bacteria，fungi，protozoa and some algae are all included in this category. Our world is populated by those invisible creatures. They are small and widely distributed，and have a close relationship with human life activities.

The size and cell type of microbes（微生物的大小和细胞类型）

Most of the bacteria and fungi are single-celled microorganisms，and even the multi-celled microbes do not have a great range of cell types. Viruses are not cells. They are genetic material surrounded by a protein coat and incapable of independent existence（Fig. 1-2）.

The classification of microbes（微生物的分类）

Prokaryotic microbes （原核微生物）

Prokaryotes are a class of primitive single-celled organisms with nuclear

microbe	approximate range of sizes	cell type
viruses	0.01~0.25μm	acellular
bacteria	0.1~10μm	prokaryote
fungi	2μm~1m	eukaryote
protozoa	2~1000μm	eukaryote
algae	1μm~ several meters	eukaryote

Fig. 1-2   The size and cell type of microbes

membranes encapsulated in bare DNA. The most common prokaryotes are bacteria. They are single-celled small individuals with simple structure, which has cell walls, but lacks organelles.

Bacteria have a few basic shapes, including spherical coccus (plural cocci, meaning berries), rod-shaped bacillus (the word is derived from the Greek "plural bacilli", meaning "a small staff"), and spiral (Fig. 1-3).

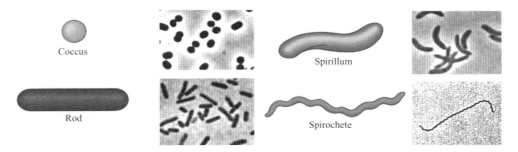

Coccus

Spirillum

Rod

Spirochete

Fig. 1-3   The shape of the bacteria

Bacteria can be divided into two major groups, Gram-positive bacteria and Gram-negative bacteria. The original distinction between Gram-positive bacteria and Gram-negative bacteria was based on a special staining procedure——the Gram stain. The cell wall of the Gram-positive bacteria has a peptidoglycan layer that is relatively thick and comprises approximately 90% of the cell wall. The cell walls of most Gram-positive bacteria also have teichoic acids (Fig. 1-4, and see colored picture).

The mechanism of Gram staining (革兰染色机理)

After the bacteria were first stained with crystal violet and mediated by iodine solution, a water-insoluble complex of crystal violet and iodine was formed in the cell wall of bacteria. Gram-positive bacteria have thicker cell walls

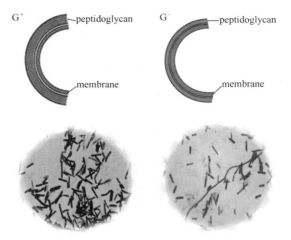

Fig. 1-4　The structure of Gram-positive and Gram-negative

and higher content of peptidoglycan. When decolorized by ethanol, the meshes shrink because of water loss. They do not contain lipids and there will be no cracks in ethanol treatment. Therefore, they can keep the crystal violet and iodine complex firmly in the wall and make it still purple. Gram-negative bacteria have thin cell walls, high lipid content and low peptidoglycan content. After decolorization with ethanol, they become colorless, and then re-dyed with red dyes such as sand yellow, which makes Gram-negative bacteria red (Fig. 1-5).

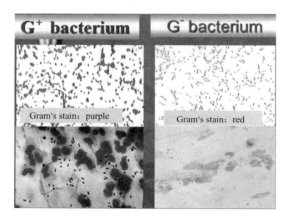

Fig. 1-5　Gram stain

Eukaryotic microbes（真核微生物）

Fungi are heterotrophic eukaryotic microorganisms. They are nonphotosynthetic and typically form reproductive spores. Mucor (class Zygomycetes) occur abun-dantly in soil and on fruits，vegetables and starchy foods. Some are used in the manufacture of cheese. Their mycelium is nonseptate，white or gray. Zygospores are produced when plus and minus strains are both present. Penicillium（class Deuteromycetes）members of them occur widely in nature. Some species cause rot or other spoilage. Some are used in industrial fermentations，and penicillin is produced by *P. notatum* and *P. chrysogenum*. Some reproduce sexually by ascospore formation. Penicillia have septate vegetative mycelium. Yeasts are usually unicellular. Yeast cells are larger than most bacteria，$1\sim5\mu$m in width and $5\sim30\mu$m or more in length. They are commonly egg-shaped. Yeasts have no flagella.

Virus（病毒）

What is a virus？（什么是病毒？）

Virus is a simple biologic viral agent that is composed of a nucleic acid core （either DNA or RNA）surrounded by a protein coat. Viruses have a wide range of shapes. A virus can have either DNA or RNA，but never both!

Diseases related to virus infection（病毒感染引起的疾病）

Viral Infections may lead to a range of problems：Damage to the liver，Hepatitis，HIV，damage to the nervous system，impairment of the immune system——HIV，cancer——leukemia，cervical cancer. Viruses spread in air，in blood，in semen，in saliva，in food，in water，on dirt，but they themselves do not move. They are particles that are infectious. They do not excrete and they do not metabolize. They simply infect and reproduce.

Reproductive Cycle of the virus（病毒的繁殖）（Fig. 1-6）

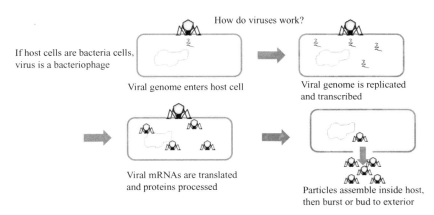

Fig. 1-6   The reproductive cycle of the virus

Vocabulary（课文词汇）

microbe 微生物

microorganism 微生物

organism 机体、生物体

virus 病毒

bacteria 细菌

fungi 真菌

Gram stain 革兰染色

mechanism 机理

Gram-negative 革兰阴性

Gram-positive 革兰阳性

prokaryotic 原核的

eukaryotic 真核的

protein 蛋白质

nucleic acid 核酸

Summary（重点小结）

1. The word microbe（microorganism）is used to describe an organism that is so small that normally it cannot be seen without the use of a microscope.

2. Bacteria can be divided into two major groups，called Gram-positive bacteria and Gram-negative bacteria. The original distinction between Gram-positive and Gram-negative was based on a special staining procedure.

3. Fungi are heterotrophic eukaryotic microorganisms.

4. Viruses are composed of a nucleic acid core（either DNA or RNA）surrounded by a protein coat.

5. Viral Infections may lead to all kinds of the diseases.

Quiz（课后检测）

Ⅰ. **Fill in the blanks according to the information about microbe.**

1. The features of the microorganism include _____、_____、_____.

2. Bacteria can be divided into _____ and _____ .

3. Viruses are composed of _____ 、 _____ .

4. Viral Infections may lead to all kinds of the _____ .

Ⅱ. **Identify the type of microbes shown in the picture below.**

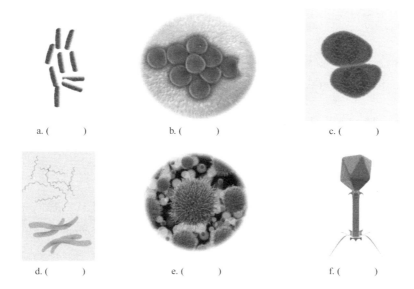

a. (   )   b. (   )   c. (   )

d. (   )   e. (   )   f. (   )

Ⅲ. **Sterile eggs are being produced and ready for infection with virus particles e. g. flu virus. The virus multiplies inside the egg cells and can be harvested at a later time. Virus is chemically/heat treated to render in non-infectious and can then be used as a vaccine. Discuss the relationship between the vaccine, microbes and the diseases according to the pictures below and pharmaceutical professional knowledge in English.**

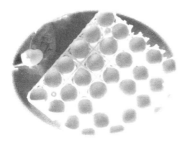   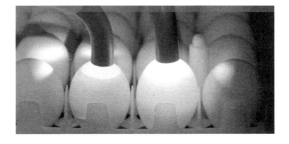

Eggs being candled to evaluate their quality: left＝healthy egg; right ＝ unhealthy egg to be removed

Discussion（问题讨论）

- Could we see the microbes around our world with the unaided eye?
- What is the difference between the bacteria and virus?
- What is the difference between the prokaryotic microbes and eukaryotic microbes?
- Did you ever get the disease related to virus infections?
- Could you identify the Gram-negative bacteria and Gram-positive bacteria?

Reading Material（延伸阅读）

SARS Virus
（严重急性呼吸道综合征病毒）

SARS virus is a variant of coronavirus and the cause of atypical pneumonia. Variant coronavirus is related to influenza virus，but it is a very unique coronavirus. The coronavirus is the culprit of the severe acute respiratory Syndrome (SARS，infectious atypical pneumonia) that raged around the world in the winter of 2002 to the spring of 2003.

By the end of 2002，there were many unexplained and life-threatening respiratory diseases in Guangdong and other places in China. Subsequently，similar cases were reported in Vietnam，Canada and Hongkong. WHO named the disease "Severe Acute Respiratory Syndrome (SARS)". Subsequently，laboratories around the world worked to discover the pathogen of the disease.

University of Hong Kong first announced the isolation of an unknown coronavirus in March 22，2003. Subsequently，a number of laboratories published research papers on the pathogen in NJEM，Lancet and other internationally renowned medical journals. The genome science center (BC Cancer Agency's Genome Sciences Center) of the BC Cancer Institute，Canada，completed the whole genome sequencing of the virus on April 12，2003. On April 16，2003，on the basis of the above research results，WHO officially declared a previously unknown coronavirus，the pathogen leading to SARS，and named it the SARS Coronavirus (SARS-CoV).

In 2013，the international research team，led by Shi Zhengli，a researcher at the Wuhan Institute of virus research，Chinese Academy of Sciences，separated a SARS like coronavirus with a high homologous SARS virus，and further confirmed that the chrysanthemum bats were the source of SARS virus.

Lesson 2　Biology of the Human Body
第二课　人体生物学

Situational Entry（情境导入）

In order to fully understand the mechanisms of human physiology，it is important to have an understanding of the chemical composition and system of the body and how its parts are put together. This will come in handy when considering the various interactions between cells and structures. The study of the human body involves anatomy and physiology. The study of the body's structure is called anatomy，the study of the body's function is known as physiology. Other studies of human body include biology，cytology，embryology，histology，endocrinology，hematology，immunology，psychology，etc. The human body is organized at different levels，starting with the cell and ending with the entire system (Fig. 2-1).

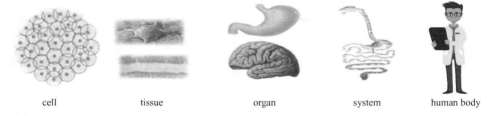

cell　　　　tissue　　　　organ　　　　system　　　　human body

Fig. 2-1　Organization of the human body

Information about human body（人体的相关知识）

Chemical elements（化学元素）

Two people of equal height and body weight may look completely different from each other because they have a different body composition. The most common chemical elements in the human body are oxygen (65.0% by mass)，carbon (18.5%)，hydrogen (9.5%)，nitrogen (3.2%)，calcium (1.5%)，and phosphorus (1. 0%). These six elements make up 99% of the mass of the human body. Potassium (0. 4%), sulfur (0. 3%), sodium (0. 2%), chlorine (0. 2%) and magnesium (0. 1%) are the next five most common elements. Other ten elements only combine for about 0. 7% of the human body's mass: iron, copper, zinc, selenium, molybdenum, fluorine, chromium, iodine, manganese, and cobalt. Trace elements that have been identified include lithium, strontium, aluminum, silicon, lead, vanadium, arsenic, and bromine (Fig. 2-2).

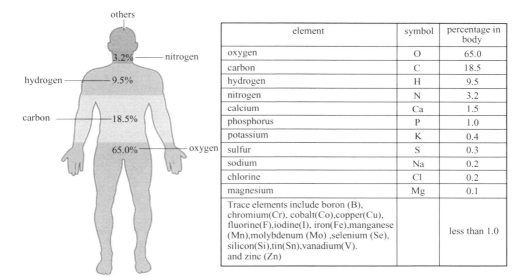

element	symbol	percentage in body
oxygen	O	65.0
carbon	C	18.5
hydrogen	H	9.5
nitrogen	N	3.2
calcium	Ca	1.5
phosphorus	P	1.0
potassium	K	0.4
sulfur	S	0.3
sodium	Na	0.2
chlorine	Cl	0.2
magnesium	Mg	0.1
Trace elements include boron (B), chromium(Cr), cobalt(Co),copper(Cu), fluorine(F),iodine(I), iron(Fe),manganese (Mn),molybdenum (Mo) ,selenium (Se), silicon(Si),tin(Sn),vanadium(V). and zinc (Zn)		less than 1.0

Fig. 2-2   The composition of human body

Oxygen is used for cellular respiration. All living organisms contain carbon, which forms the basis organic molecules of the body. Carbon is the second most abundant element in the human body, accounting for 18. 5% of body weight. All organic molecules (fats, proteins, carbohydrates, nucleic acids) contain carbon. Hydrogen accounts for 9. 5% of the mass of the human body. Hydrogen is also important in energy production and use. The H^+ can be used as a hydrogen ion or proton pump to produce ATP and regulate numerous chemical reactions. All organic molecules contain hydrogen in addition to carbon. Approximately 3. 2% of the mass of the human body is nitrogen. Calcium is used to give the skeletal system rigidity and strength. Calcium is found in bones and teeth. The Ca^{2+} ion is important for muscle function. Calcium accounts for 1. 5% of human body weight. About 1. 2% to 1. 5% of your body consists of phosphorus. Phosphorus is important for bone structure and is part of the primary energy molecule in the body, ATP or adenosine triphosphate. Most of the phosphorus in the body is in bones and teeth. Potassium makes up 0.2% to 0.35% of the adult human body. Potassium is an important mineral in all cells. It functions as an electrolyte and is particularly important for conducting electrical impulses and for muscle contraction. Sulfur's abundance is 0.20% to 0.25% in the human body. Sulfur is an important component of amino acids and proteins. It presents in keratin, a type of protein that is a basic component of skin, hair, and nails. Sodium is an important electrolyte in the body. It is an important component of cellular fluids and is needed for the transmission of nerve impulses. It helps regulate fluid volume, temperature, and blood pressure. The metal magnesium comprises about 0.05% of human body weight. Magnesium is important for numerous biochemical reactions. It helps regulate heartbeat, blood pressure, and blood glucose levels. It is needed to support proper immune system, muscle and nerve function.

Cells (细胞)

The average adult human body is estimated to have ten trillion to one hundred trillion cells. There are a wide variety of types of cells, and they differ in size, shape, and function. Among the types of cells are bone cells, blood cells, nerve cells, muscle cells, stomach cells, and so forth. Red blood cells carry oxygen, bone cells form the skeleton of the body, nerve cells carry electrical signals, and muscle cells move the bones. Stomach cells secrete acids to digest food, while cells in the intestines absorb nutrients.

Tissues (组织)

Tissues are collections of similar cells that perform a specialized function. The human body has four primary tissue types, such as muscle tissue, nerve tissue, epithelial tissue and connective tissue.

Organs (器官)

An organ is a group of two or more different kinds of tissues that work together to perform a specific function or group of functions. Examples of organs include the heart, lung, brain, eye, stomach, spleen, pancreas, kidneys, liver, intestines, uterus, bladder, and so forth. The largest organ in the human body is the skin.

Systems（系统）

A group of organs functioning as a unit is called a system, or organ system. For example, the stomach, small intestine, liver, and pancreas are part of the digestive system, and the kidneys, bladder, and connecting tubes constitute the urinary system. The principal parts of some of these systems are described below (Fig. 2-3).

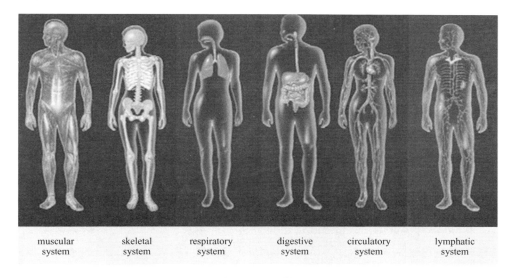

| muscular system | skeletal system | respiratory system | digestive system | circulatory system | lymphatic system |

Fig. 2-3   The system of human body

The skeletal system is made of bones, joints between bones, and cartilage. Your skeleton has five major functions. It provides shape and support, enables you to move, protects your internal organs, produces blood cells, and stores certain materials until your body needs them. There are 206 bones in the human skeleton. They have various shapes——long, short, cube-shaped, flat, and irregular. A joint is a place in the body where two bones come together. Joints allow bones to move in different ways. Cartilage is a more flexible material than bone. As an infant, much of your skeleton was cartilage. By the time you stop growing, most of the cartilage will have been replaced with hard bone tissue. It serves as a protective, cushioning layer where bones come together. It also connects the ribs to the breastbone and provides a structural base for the nose and the external ear.

The muscular system allows the body to move, and its contractions produce heat, which helps maintain a constant body temperature. Your body has three types of muscle tissue——skeletal muscle, smooth muscle, and cardiac muscle. Cardiac muscles are involuntary muscles found only in the heart. Cardiac muscles do not get tired. Smooth muscles are called involuntary muscles because they work with your conscious effort. The muscles that are under your direct control are called voluntary muscles. Smiling and turning the pages in a book are actions of voluntary muscles. The muscles that are not under your conscious control are called involuntary muscles. Your colon is lined with smooth muscle, and your heart is comprised of cardiac muscle that works automatically pumping blood around your body.

Your digestive system is like a complicated chemical processing plant and performs many functions. It breaks down food into molecules that the body can absorb and passes these molecules into the blood to be carried throughout the body. It can eliminate solid wastes from the body. Digestion begins in your mouth with the action of your teeth and tongue (mechanical digestion) and your salivary glands (chemical digestion). The salivary glands produce enzymes that are mixed with the food, breaking down the starches (淀粉). Peristalsis (蠕动) is the muscular action that moves the food through the esophagus (食道) and into your stomach after you swallow. The food moves into your stomach, which contains chemicals such as hydrochloric acid and pepsin. Pepsin breaks proteins, and other enzymes break down fat. Your stomach gradually releases these materials into the upper small intestine (duodenum), where digestion is completed. In the small intestines all the nutrients are absorbed, leaving indigestible wastes behind. These wastes pass into the large intestines, where water is removed. Then the wastes are stored in the rectum until they are released by the anus.

Your respiratory system moves oxygen from the outside environment into your body. It also removes carbon dioxide and water from your body. Pneumonia is an inflammation or infection of the lungs most commonly caused by a bacteria or virus. Pneumonia can also be caused by inhaling vomit or other foreign substances. The respiratory and circulatory systems work together and form the cardiopulmonary system, which is an integral connection between the heart and lungs.

Your lymphatic system filters out organisms that cause disease. There are two major kinds of lymphocytes——T cells and B cells. A major function of T cells is to identify pathogens by recognizing their antigens. Antigens are molecules that the immune system recognizes as either part of your body, or as coming from outside your body. B cells produce chemicals called antibodies. It is also important for the distribution of fluids and nutrients in the body, because it drains excess fluids and protein so that tissues do not swell up.

Your Immune System includes immune organs and immune tissues, immunocytes, and immune molecules. It is a network of cells, tissues, and organs that work together to defend the body against attacks by "foreign" invaders. These invaders are primarily microbes (germs)——tiny, infection-causing organisms such as bacteria, viruses parasites, and fungi. The key to a healthy immune system is its remarkable ability to distinguish between the body's own cells-self and foreign cells-nonself. Adaptive and innate immunity does not operate independently. They function as a highly interactive and cooperative system, producing a total response more effective than either could alone.

Your integumentary system is your skin. The skin is a complete layer that protects the inner structures of the body, and it is the largest organ. Your skin covers your body and prevents the loss of water. It protects the body from injury and infection. The skin also helps to regulate body temperature, eliminate wastes, gather information about the environment, and produce vitamin D. The skin is organized into two main layers, the epidermis and the dermis.

Vocabulary（课文词汇）

oxygen 氧气
carbon 碳
hydrogen 氢
organic 有机的
molecule 分子
calcium 钙
potassium 钾
nitrogen 氮

phosphorus 磷

magnesium 镁

sulfur 硫

sodium 钠

chlorine 氯

skeletal system 骨骼系统

muscular system 肌肉系统

digestive system 消化系统

respiratory system 呼吸系统

lymphatic system 淋巴系统

immune system 免疫系统

integumentary system 皮肤系统

Summary（重点小结）

1. Most of the human body is made up of water，with cells consisting of 65%～90% water by weight.

2. In the small intestines all the nutrients are absorbed，leaving indigestible wastes behind.

3. The muscular system allows the body to move，and its contractions produce heat，which helps maintain a constant body temperature.

4. The respiratory and circulatory systems work together and form the cardio-pulmonary system，which is an integral connection between the heart and lungs.

5. Your immune system includes immune organs and immune tissues，immunocytes，immune molecules.

6. The skin is organized into two main layers，the epidermis and the dermis.

Quiz（课后检测）

Ⅰ. **Fill in the blanks according to the information about human body.**

1. _____ enters through the mouth，where chewing and saliva start to break it up and make it easier to _____ .

2. The _____ system distributes needed materials and removes unneeded ones.

3. _____ is used to give the skeletal system its rigidity and strength. _____ is found in bones and teeth.

4. _____ is important for bone structure and is part of the primary energy molecule in the body.

Ⅱ. **Please label the parts of your system on your handout. Can you describe the path that air takes as it enters and leaves your body?**

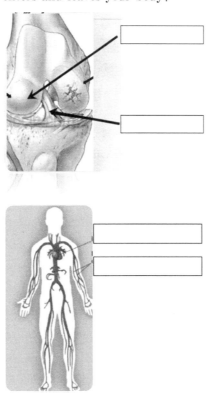

Discussion（问题讨论）

• If two people could have the same body composition when they have the equal height and body weight?

• Which element is the most abundant in the human body?

• What is the second most abundant element in the human body?

• Which system provides support and protection for the soft tissues and the organs of the body and to provide points of attachment for the muscles that move the body?

- How many bones are there in the human skeleton?
- What major tasks does your digestive system help you accomplish?
- How does your immune system work?

Reading Material（延伸阅读）

How does human body biological clock work?
（人体生物钟是如何工作的？）

We all know that the normal human daily cycle of activity is of some $7 \sim 8$ hours' sleep alternation with some $16 \sim 17$ hours' wakefulness. And, the sleep normally coincides with the hours of darkness. Our concern is how easily and to what extent this cycle can be modified. The question is no mere academic one. The ease, for example, with which people can change from working in the day to working at night is a question of growing importance in an industry where automation calls for the round-the-clock working of machines. It normally takes five to seven days for a person to adapt to a reversed routine of sleep and wakefulness, sleeping during the day and working at night. Unfortunately, it is often the case in an industry that shifts are changed every week. A person may work from 12:00 midnight to 8:00 a.m. one week, 8:00 a.m. to 4:00 p.m. the next, and 4:00 p.m. to 12:00 midnight the third and so on. This means that no sooner has he got used to one routine that has to change to another, so that much of his time is spent neither working nor sleeping very efficiently.

The only real solution appears to be to hand over the night shift to a number of permanent night workers. An interesting study of the domestic life and health of night-shift workers was carried out by Brown in 1957. She found a high incidence of disturbed sleep and other disorders among those on alternating day and night shifts, but no abnormal occurrence of these phenomena among those on permanent night work.

This latter system appears to be the best long-term policy, meanwhile something may be done to relieve the strains of alternate day and night work by selecting those people who can adapt quickly to the changes of routine. One way of knowing when a person has adapted is by measuring his body temperature. People engaged in normal daytime work will have a high temperature during the hours of wakefulness and a low one at night. When they change to night work, the pattern will only gradually change to match the new routine, and the speed with which it does so parallels the adaptation of the body as a whole, particularly in terms of performance. Therefore, by taking body temperature at intervals of two hours throughout the period of wakefulness it can be seen how quickly a person can adapt to a reversed routine, and this could be used as a basis for selection. So far, however, such a form of selection does not seem to have been applied in practice.

Lesson 3   Human Health and Diseases
第三课   人体健康与疾病

Situational Entry（情境导入）

Everyone in modern society faces the fierce competition. More and more people are in the sub-health state. Sub-health suggests a grey health status，"somewhere" between health and disease. Sub-health is a critical state that people do not have a clear symptom of any disease. When the human body has been in the sub-health state for a long time，it can lead to the occurrence of diseases，such as chronic disease（diabetes，hypertension）（Fig. 3-1）. According to a recent survey，sub-health is afflicting 60％ of middle-aged and elderly. And females are more susceptible（易患病的）to sub-health than males. The sub-health condition will negatively affect China's long-term development and sustained progress if not handled timely and properly. Non-communicable diseases（NCDs）kill more than 36 million people each year. Nearly 80％ of NCD deaths，estimated 29 million，occur in low-and middle-income countries. Thus we will discuss the human health and diseases that you need to know on this topic.

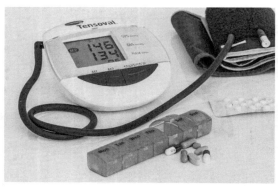
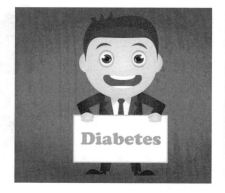

Fig. 3-1   The hypertension and diabetes

Information about Human health and diseases（人体健康和疾病的相关知识）

WHO（World Health Organization）definition of health（世界卫生组织关于健康的定义）

Health is a state of complete physical，mental and social well-being and not merely the absence of disease or infirmity.

What is a disease?（什么是疾病?）

Then what is a disease? It may be defined as a condition that impairs the proper function of the body or one of its parts. Every living thing，both plants and animals，can succumb to a disease. People，for example，are often infected by tiny bacteria. But bacteria，in turn，can be infected by even more minute viruses.

Hundreds of different diseases exist. Each has its own particular set of symptoms and signs，clues that enable a physician to diagnose the problem. A symptom is something a patient can detect，such as fever，bleeding，or pain. A sign is something a doctor can detect，such as a swollen blood vessel or an enlarged internal body organ. Diseases can be classified differently. For instance，an epidemic disease is one that strikes many person in a community. When it strikes the same region year after year it is an endemic disease. An acute disease has a quick onset and runs a short course. An acute heart attack，for example，often hits without warning and can be quickly fatal. A chronic disease has a slow onset and runs a sometimes years-long course. The gradual onset and long course of rheumatic fever make it a chronic ailment. Between the acute and chronic，another type is called subacute.

Acute disease and a chronic disease（急性病和慢性病）

Many individuals confuse the difference between an acute disease and a chronic disease. An acute disease lasts for just a short time but can begin rapidly and have intense symptoms. By contrast，a chronic disease produces symptoms that last for three months or more (Fig. 3-2).

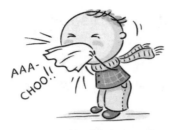 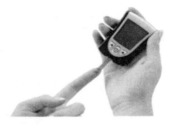

(a) A season cold and flu is a cute disease   (b) Diabetes is a chronnic disease

Fig. 3-2   The acute disease and chronic disease

Acute disease（急性病）

Often，people are confused about what constitutes an acute disease. They believe that an acute disease is always severe. In reality，an acute disease can be mild，severe or even fatal. The term "acute" does not indicate the severity of the disease. Instead，it indicates how long the disease lasts and how quickly it develops. Examples of acute diseases include colds，influenza and strep throat. Some acute diseases might resolve themselves without significant medical attention or treatment. For example，an individual might recover from influenza at home without taking prescription medications or requiring the care of a physician. Pneumonia，on the other hand，is an acute disease that often requires medical care and prescription medication. Frequently，hospitalization is required as well.

Chronic disease（慢性病）

Chronic，non-communicable diseases（NCDs）are steadily increasing around the world. They are also known as chronic diseases，and not passed from person to person. They are of long duration and generally slow progression. The four main types of non-communicable diseases are cardiovascular diseases（like heart attacks and stroke），cancers，chronic respiratory diseases（such as chronic obstructed pulmonary disease and asthma）and diabetes. The prevalence rate of chronic diseases is higher in low-income and middle-income countries than it is in high-income countries，and continues to rise.

Here are some examples of common chronic diseases：

disease	example
cardiovascular disease	heart attack，stroke，PAD
pulmonary disease	asthma，COPD，emphysema
diabetes	neuropathies，CAD

neuromuscular disorders	multiple sclerosis，Parkinsons
musculoskeletal conditions	arthritis
cancer	breast，prostate，leukemia
renal disease	kidney failure，CAD
immunological	AIDS

The report on China's health management and health industry development (2018) shows that the number of patients with chronic diseases in China was about 300 million. 50% of the patients were under 65 years old. The incidence of deaths from chronic diseases accounted for 85.3% and 79.5% of the total deaths respectively in urban and rural areas of China. Among them，9.4%，3.9% and 3.4% were associated with hypertension，high cholesterol and diabetes，respectively. Chronic diseases have become the harmful killer that endangering the health of Chinese resident.

Chronic diseases often require the care of medical professionals and the use of prescription medications. Sometimes，hospitalization is required as well. For example，an individual who has diabetes might need to see a doctor on a regular basis and take prescribed medications. An individual who has kidney disease might require professional medical care，medication and dialysis. Frequently，medical intervention might make an individual who has a chronic disease more comfortable or might reduce the symptoms，but chronic diseases often cannot be cured.

Vocabulary（课文词汇）

symptom 症状

severity 严重

diagnose 诊断

endemic 地方性的，地方病

cancer 癌症

AIDS 获得性免疫缺陷综合征，艾滋病

acute disease 急性病

chronic disease 慢性病

asymptomatic 无症状的

Parkinsons 帕金森

collaboration 合作

infectious disease 传染性疾病

leukemia 白血病

obesity 肥胖

diabetes 糖尿病

pulmonary disease 肺疾病

arthritis 关节炎

multiple sclerosis（MS）多发性硬化

cardiovascular disease 心血管疾病

breast cancer 乳腺癌

prostate 前列腺癌

Summary（重点小结）

1. Health is a state of complete physical，mental and social well-being and not merely the absence of disease or infirmity.

2. A chronic disease has a slow onset and runs a sometimes years-long course.

3. An acute disease has a quick onset and runs a short course. An acute heart attack，for example，often hits without warning and can be quickly fatal.

4. The four main types of non-communicable diseases are cardiovascular diseases（like heart attacks and stroke），cancers，chronic respiratory diseases（such as chronic obstructed pulmonary disease and asthma）and diabetes.

Quiz（课后检测）

Fill in the blanks according to the information about disease.

1. Chronic diseases often require the care of _____ and the use of _____ medications.

2. Common acute diseases include colds，_____ and _____ .

3. Health is a state of complete _____ 、_____ and social well-being and not merely the absence of _____ or _____ .

4. _____ diseases are not passed from person to person.

Discussion（问题讨论）

• According to data from recent surveys，there is an increasing trend of chronic，mental and psychiatric illnesses．Talk about your opinion on the chronic disease.

- What is the difference between the chronic disease and the acute disease?
- What should you do when you got a chronic disease?
- What should you do when you got an acute disease?

Reading Material（延伸阅读）

Obvious warnings from your body
（来自身体的警报）

The body speaks volumes about what ails it，from obvious warnings like a fever that accompanies an infection to subtle clues like losing hair on the toes，which can be an early sign of vascular disease.

Some signs that seem alarming may actually be harmless. Bright-red stools are more likely to come from eating beets than from intestinal bleeding．But some that seem minor can warn of a serious disorder．Small yellow bumps on the eyelid，for instance，may be fatty deposits that signal high cholesterol，which in turn raises the risk of heart disease.

"If I see a patient with a horizontal line through the middle of the fingernails，I'll ask what happened three months ago. Were they horribly ill or did someone die? They think I'm brilliant." says Dr. Parsons．The markings，called Beau's lines，sometimes appear when the body is particularly stressed． "Your body is busy，so your nails take a little break and then start growing a-gain," Dr. Parsons says.

Nails tell other tales as well．White nail beds，the skin underneath the nail，can signify anemia．Nails that are white near the cuticle and red or brown near the tip can be a sign of kidney disease．Irregularly shaped brown or blue spots in the nail bed can be melanomas．Fingertips that are blue or clubbed can be a sign of lung disease．Although generally，there would be more significant signs as well.

Many of the same signs occur in toenails．But the feet are critical for other reasons． "Feet tell you a huge amount about the health of the circulation," says Dr. Denman，the Duke nursing instructor． "The first place that vascular disease can show up is where the blood vessels are the smallest and the farthest away from the heart. "

Circulatory problems can manifest themselves as numbness and tingle in the feet; so can peripheral neuropathy, or damage to the nerves that often begins in the extremities. Both are signs of uncontrolled diabetes. With circulation compromised, even a minor scratch or sore on the feet can become infected easily; lack of sensation can make it easy to ignore, and gangrene can set in, requiring amputation. That's why people with diabetes are urged to check their feet every day for any kind of scratch or lesion.

Lesson 4   How does the Body Fight Back Disease?
第四课   人体如何对抗疾病？

Situational Entry（情境导入）

Human body lives in a world where many other living things compete for food and places to breed. Antigen（substances could harm the body if they ever entered it，ranging from bacteria and pollen to transplanted organ），such as the pathogenic organisms，or pathogens，often broadly called germs，that cause many diseases are able to invade the human body and use its cells and fluids for their own needs（Fig. 4-1）.

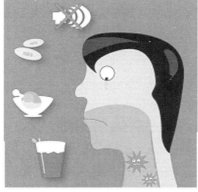
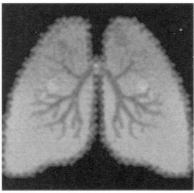

Fig. 4-1   Antigen invade the human body

Ordinarily, the body's defense system can ward off these invaders. Pathogenic organisms can enter the body in various ways. Some, such as these that cause the common cold, pneumonia, and tuberculosis are breathed in. Others, such as those that cause hepatitis, colitis, cholera, and typhoid fever get in the body through contaminated food, water or utensils. Insects can spread disease by acting as vectors, or carriers. Flies can carry germs from human waste or other tainted materials to food and beverages. Germs may also enter the body through the bite of a mosquito, louse, or other insect vector.

Information about immune to disease （疾病免疫的相关知识）

The body's defense system （人体免疫系统）

In order to fight the disease, the human body has established a complex defense system. First, this system is to protect the human body from viruses, bacteria, mycoplasma and other pathogenic microorganisms. Second, it is to clean up the waste after metabolism in time, to clean up the battlefield after the battle of human and pathogenic microbes, to eliminate the mutant human cells. Third, it is to repair the injured organs and tissues and let them restore normal function. The human body's defense system consists of three levels. They are physical barriers, non-specific immune systems and specific immune systems. These defense systems are made up of system level. After pathogen conquered the first barrier, they immediately faced second barriers. This multi-layered system makes it possible for humans to survive thousands of pathogenic bacteria every day.

How does the body deal with the invasion of the pathogen? （人体如何应对入侵的病原体?）

The human body's Great Wall, the skin and mucous membrane of the skin constructed the most outer natural barrier. The human body only exchanges with the outside world through the mouth, the nasal cavity, the urethra, and the anus to complete the energy metabolism. Meanwhile, the existence of these ports also provides a way of invasion for pathogenic microorganisms. The skin consists of multi-layer flat cells that block the passage of pathogens. Only when the skin is damaged can the pathogen invade. Many layers of flat cells in the skin are dead cells and glia cells. Viruses have to invade the human body through living cells and reach the corresponding target cells. So the virus, such as influenza, measles and chickenpox, can not be transmitted through the whole skin. The sweat glands of the skin secrete lactic acid, which is acidic and is not conducive to the growth of bacteria. Fatty acids secreted by sebaceous glands can kill bacteria and fungi.

Although there are only monolayer columnar cells in the mucosa, the mechanical barrier is not as good as the skin, there are many kinds of weapons in the mucosa. There are epithelial cells on the surface of the respiratory tract. These epithelial cells not only have cilia structure but also secrete mucus. The surface of the respiratory tract of a healthy person can produce about 100 milliliters of mucus every day. Mucus not only facilitates the movement of cilia, but also adheres to the pathogenic microorganism and impedes its entry into the cell. The cilia of the epithelial cells has an active swinging action, which moves in a certain direction so that the pathogens in mucus and mucus itself move to the throat, and they are discharged through coughing and swallowing. In some of the airway mucus is swimming with some mobile units (phagocytes and white blood cells), which can eat pathogens or restrict the spread of pathogens at any time. The anterior part of the nasal cavity has nasal hair, and the nasal hair is interwoven into a large net to trap most of the dust and larger bacteria; the cilia and mucus in the back of the nasal cavity can stick to most of the pathogens and remove the pathogens by sneezing and blowing nose.

The digestive tract is also a difficult barrier to overpass. Only the most resistant pathogens can achieve infection through the digestive tract. The first pass of the pathogen is the mouth. Oral saliva contains saliva amylase and lysozymes. Saliva amylase can chemically breaks down carbohydrates into simpler compounds. Lysozymes can efficiently decompose bacteria. Swallowing can also shorten the retention time of pathogens in the mouth, so that pathogens do not have enough time to reproduce. The pathogen will face the attack of gastric acid after fluke passing through it. Gastric acid can almost kill most of the microorganisms in food. There are many proteases in the stomach, which have the best activity under the action of gastric acid to degrade protein in food and, of course, decompose the protein of the pathogenic microorganism. The duodenum has a large number of digestive enzymes from the pancreas and bile from the liver. It has a good dissolution effect on the protein shell and lipids of the pathogen, which can quickly kill these pathogenic microorganisms. In addition, hundreds of trillions of beneficial bacteria have been distributed in the intestines, which have already been carved up and can compete with pathogenic bacteria. Intestinal tract and urethra excrete harmful bacteria and substances rapidly through regular excretion.

The human field army, the pathogenic microbes that are exposed to the human body in the natural immune system——are inestimable astronomical figures. We can't rely on the Great Wall only to prevent the invasion of pathogens. The main function of this physical barrier is to minimize the number of pathogens. The pathogen is very cunning and will not be frightened by the tall walls. The pathogen will invade the human body through various channels for survival. If they do not infect humans or other animals, they can not survive and reproduce, which will lead to the death of the family. Pathogens coexist with human beings, and they will fight with human beings for a long time. In addition to the barrier of skin and mucous membrane, the body also has a set of immune systems, including innate immunity and acquired immunity. It is a defense system that resists pathogenic microorganisms. This system is made up of immune organs, immune cells and immune molecules.

The natural immune system consists of two main military types. One is the phagocytic system, and the other is the immunoglobulin system. When the pathogen invades the human body, macrophages are the first ones to rush forward. In the age of peace, the main function of macrophages is to cruise in tissue to collect the body's garbage, such as the cell fragments of death, because a large number of cells die every day due to the metabolism of the human body. Once the pathogenic microorganism passes through the first barrier, the macrophages swallowed them up without mercy. But in most of the cases, the macrophages can only deal with a small number of pathogens and play a more important role in notifying enemy conditions. When the enemy is tough, it will quickly report to the command and mobilize the field forces, white cells (the powerful phagocytes, including neutrophils and mononuclear cells). That's why when we get sick, the doctor will give us a white blood cell examination. If it is bacterial infection, the white blood cell number will rise. So many people think that white blood cells are bad and it causes illness. In fact, this is the result, not the reason. White blood cells are the warriors who fight against the bacteria in the human body and fight against the enemy until they die. In the course of fighting with the enemy, a variety of hydrolase released by lysosomes in white cells can also destroy adjacent normal tissue cells, causing adverse immune pathological damage to the human body.

Vocabulary（课文词汇）

pathogenic 病原的、致病的

mycoplasma 支原体

glia 神经胶质的

secrete 分泌

monolayer 单层

mucosa 黏膜

protease 蛋白酶

phagocyte 吞噬作用

cruise 巡游、巡航

gastric acid 胃酸

macrophage 巨噬细胞

hydrolase 水解酶

neutrophils cell 中性粒细胞

pathological 病理的

Summary（重点小结）

1. The human body's defense system consists of three levels. They are physical barriers, non-specific immune systems and specific immune systems.

2. The human body's Great Wall, the skin and mucous membrane of the skin constructed the most outer natural barrier.

3. The natural immune system consists of two main military types. One is

the phagocytic system，and the other is the immunoglobulin system.

4. In the age of peace，the main function of macrophages is to cruise in tissue to collect the body's garbage，such as the cell fragments of death，because a large number of cells die every day due to the metabolism of the human body.

5. White blood cells are the warriors who fight against the bacteria in the human body and fight against the enemy until they die.

Quiz（课后检测）

Ⅰ. **Fill in the blanks according to the information about immune to disease.**

1. In order to fight the disease，the human body has established a complex _____ .

2. When the pathogen invades the human body，_____ are the first ones to rush forward.

3. _____ can almost kill most of the microorganisms in food.

4. The main function of macrophages is to _____ in tissue to collect the body's garbage，such as the cell fragments of death.

Ⅱ. **Analyze the role of antibody according to the following diagram features.**

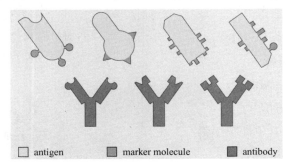

□ antigen   ▨ marker molecule   ■ antibody

Discussion（问题讨论）

- How many levels do the human body's defense system consists of?
- What is the function of the macrophages?
- What is the natural immune system?
- What are the field forces of the body?
- What does the white blood cell do if our body is infected by the bacteria?

Reading Material（延伸阅读）

How many fruits and vegetables does the body need?
（身体需要多少水果和蔬菜？）

Experts say eating a range of fruit and vegetables is the best，as part of a balanced diet，to protect against illness. Research suggests eating at least seven portions of fruit and vegetables a day is more effective at preventing disease than the government's current five-a-day recommendation.

Is five-a-day enough? Yes. People should eat at least five portions of fruit and vegetables a day，the government says. The advice is based on World Health Organization guidelines，which are 25 years old. Dieticians say eating five a day is enough to get the protective benefits of fruit and vegetable，although eating more may be additionally beneficial.

What counts as a portion? Fruit juice counts towards one portion of the recommended five portions per day. For an adult，a minimum of 400g of fruits and vegetables should be eaten every day or five portions of 80g. The amount varies for children，based on activity levels and age，but a rough guide is that one portion should fit in the palm of their hand. Fruit and vegetables do not have to be eaten on their own and can be cooked in dishes such as soups，stews or pasta meals.

Do tinned fruit and fruit juice count? Yes. But juice should be unsweetened，and only counts as one portion a day，as it contains less fibre than whole fruits and vegetables. Fruit must be tinned in natural juice，or water，with no added sugar or salt，and not in syrup，which lots of fruit are. Beans and pulses also count，but again only as one portion as they contain fewer nutrients than other fruits and vegetables. Smoothies may count towards more than one portion if they contain all the edible pulped fruit or vegetable，and depending on their ingredients. Recommendations include frozen fruit and vegetables，and dried fruit，such as currants，dates，sultanas，and figs. Those in ready-meals and shop-bought pasta sauces，soups and puddings are also included，but advice urges "only to have them occasionally" or in small amounts，as they are often high in salt，sugar and fat.

What about potatoes? Potatoes do not count towards one of the five-a-day， but sweet potatoes do. Potatoes are not one of the five-a-day items. This is because they mainly contribute starch to a healthy diet, which is a good source of energy and helps digestion. They are classified in the same group as bread or pasta by the government. Skins should be left on when cooking as they are a good source of fibre.

But sweet potatoes, parsnips, swedes, and turnips do count as five-a-day foods, as they are usually eaten as well as the starchy bit of the meal.

Unit 2

Basic Theory of Production Technique for Pharmacy
第二单元 药品生产技术理论基础

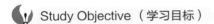

Study Objective（学习目标）

1. Grasping the pharmaceutical English terms.
2. Learning how to translate pharmaceutical English.
3. Getting familiar with the important knowledge of production technique for pharmacy.

Lesson 5　Pharmacology
第五课　药理学

Situational Entry（情境导入）

Side effects can occur when commencing，decreasing/increasing dosages，or ending a drug or medication regimen（Fig. 5-1）. The process of new drug research can be roughly divided into three stages：preclinical research，clinical research and post-marketing monitoring. Pharmacochemistry and pharmacology are branches of preclinical study. The pharmacochemistry focuses on the pharmaceutical process route，physicochemical properties and quality control standards. The pharmacology includes pharmacodynamics and pharmacokinetics. In

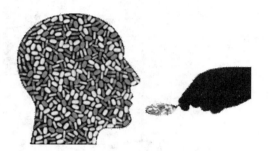

Fig. 5-1   Scientific，rational and safe medication

order to ensure the safety，effectiveness and controllability of the medication，preclinical pharmacological research plays an important role in the new drug evaluation system. Pharmacological research data is of great value to the transition from experimental research to clinical application of new drugs.

Information about pharmacology（药理学相关知识）

What is pharmacology?（什么是药理学？）

Pharmacology is the study of the action and effects of drugs on living systems and the interaction of drugs with living systems，which is divided into pharmacodynamics and pharmacokinetics. Pharmacodynamics is the study of how a drug affects an organism，whereas pharmacokinetics is the study of how the organism affects the drug. Both of them influence dosing，benefit，and adverse effects（Fig. 5-2）.

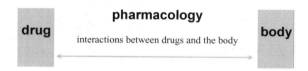

Fig. 5-2   What is pharmacology

Introduction to pharmacodynamics（药效动力学简介）

Pharmacodynamics is a branch of pharmacology，which studies the action of drugs on the physiology or pathology of the body. Pharmacodynamics places particular emphasis on dose-response relationship，that is，the relationship between drug concentration and effect.

The action of drugs（药物的作用）

The action of drugs on human physiological functions is complicated. There are two basic actions that make human physiological function enhanced or weakened，which are called excitation or inhibition. The excitation refers to an increase of the function caused by a drug. Inhibition means reducing the body function and activity. For example，the central nervous system can be stimulated by the central stimulants and body's functional activity is enhanced while general anesthetics can inhibit the central nervous system. However，the excitatory or inhibitory effect from the drug is often multi-faceted，depending on the organs the drug acts on. For example，caffeine can make the heart excited，while make the vasodilation system relaxed.

The mode of drug action（药物的作用方式）

Drug action in the local area is called local action. Aluminum hydroxide can neutralize gastric acid is one example of local action. Systemic action or absorption means drugs are distributed to tissues and organs after absorbed into the blood. Antipyretic effect of oral aspirin is a good example.

Different tissues and organs in the body have different sensitivity to drugs. Most drugs have a significant effect only on one tissue or organ at the treatment dose，and have no effect on other tissues or organs，which is called selectivity of drug action. The selectivity of drug action can theoretically be the basis of drug classification and can be used as the basis of clinical drug selection.

Drug action shows duality，that is，drugs can not only have therapeutic effects on the body，but also produce adverse reactions. Pharmacodynamics focuses on the basic action of drugs and the duality of drug action.

Structure-activity relationship of drugs（药物的构效关系）

The pharmacological specificity of many drugs is closely related to its unique chemical structure，which is called structure-activity relationship（SAR）. Similar drugs can bind to the same receptor or enzyme and produce similar or opposite effects，such as morphine and codeine，which are similar in structure and have analgesic effect.

Dose-effect relationship of drugs（药物的量效关系）

Within a certain range，the drug effect is positively correlated with the concentration on the target site，and the latter is determined by the drug dose or the drug concentration in blood. This is called the dose-effect relationship. The effects of drugs can be measured quantitatively, such as heart rate, blood pressure, respiratory rate, urine volume, blood sugar concentration, cell count, etc. This can provide evidence for new drug development. The occurrence of drug adverse reactions is related to the drug dosage. Side effects occur at therapeutic doses, and toxic reactions occur at high doses.

Introduction to pharmacokinetics（药物代谢动力学简介）

Pharmacokinetics mainly studies the dynamic changes of drugs *in vivo*, including the process of drugs *in vivo* and the rate of changes of drugs *in vivo* over time.

The process of drugs *in vivo* includes absorption, distribution, transformation and excretion. The drug must undergo multiple transmembrane transportation to complete the process of drugs *in vivo*.

Passage of a drug through a membrane（药物的跨膜转运）

The cell is contained within a membrane. The membrane is made up of a thin layer called the phospholipid bilayer. It has two layers of phospholipid molecules with phosphate heads on the surfaces and lipid (oil) tails inside (Fig. 5-3).

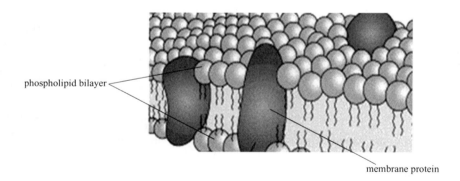

phospholipid bilayer

membrane protein

Fig. 5-3   The structure of the cell membrane

The transmembrane transport of drugs includes passive transport and active transport. Passive transport is the movement of molecules down their concentration gradient. It goes from high to low concentration, in order to maintain equilibrium in the cells. It does not require energy, including simple diffusion, filtration and easy diffusion. Active transport requires chemical energy because it is the movement of biochemicals from areas of lower concentration to areas of higher concentration.

The process of drugs in the body（药物的体内过程）

The drug enters the body from the place of administration and produces a pharmacological effect，which involves four basic process，absorption，distribution，metabolism，excretion（Fig. 5-4）.

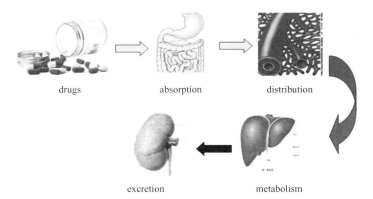

drugs   absorption   distribution

excretion   metabolism

Fig. 5-4   The process of drugs in the body

Absorption——Absorption is the transportation of the drug from the site of administration to the general circulation. Except direct injection into the blood vessels，other routes of administration involve the transport of cell membrane.

Distribution——Distribution refers to movement of the drug from the systemic circulation to tissues. The drug needs to be distributed to the site of action in sufficient concentration to generate the therapeutic action.

Metabolism——Drugs require metabolism before action. Drug metabolism occurs largely in the liver but can also occur in the kidneys，lungs，skin，and gastrointestinal tract.

Excretion——The bloodstream carries drugs from the site of absorption to the target site and also to sites of metabolism or excretion，such as the liver，the kidneys，and in some cases the lungs.

Vocabulary（课文词汇）

pharmacology 药理学

pharmacodynamics 药效动力学

pharmacokinetics 药代动力学

mechanism 机制

excitatory 兴奋的

stimulants 兴奋剂

vasodilation 血管舒张

local action 局部作用

transmembrane 跨膜的

symptomatic 有症状的

phospholipid 磷脂

biofilm 生物膜

general action 全身作用

dissemination 传播、侵染

bilayer 双层

polarity 极性

biotransformation 生物转化

excretion 排泄

Summary（重点小结）

1. Pharmacology includes pharmacodynamics and pharmacokinetics.

2. Pharmacodynamics mainly studies the action and mechanism of drugs on the organism.

3. Drug action in the local area is called local action，such as aluminum hydroxide can neutralize gastric acid. Systemic action or absorption means drugs are distributed to all the tissues and organs after drugs are absorbed into the blood. Antipyretic effect of oral aspirin is a good example.

4. Transmembrane transportation of drugs includes passive transport and active transport.

5. The drugs that enter the body produce pharmacologic effects through the delivery site. It includes four basic process，absorption，distribution，metabolism，excretion. This is called the process of drugs in the body.

6. Pharmacodynamics places particular emphasis on dose-response relationships，that is，the relationships between drug concentration and effect.

Quiz（课后检测）

Ⅰ. **Fill in the blanks.**

1. _____ is the transportation of the drug from the site of administration to the general circulation.

2. Pharmacology includes _____ and _____ .

3. The transmembrane transport of drugs includes _____ and _____ .

4. Drug metabolism occurs largely in the liver but can also occur in the _____ , _____ , skin, and _____ .

Ⅱ. **Analyze the following case and give a reasonable explanation according to the knowledge of pharmacology.**

Li Mou，a 43-year-old woman，had trouble sleeping at night in February. She woke up four to six times a night. Sometimes it was difficult to fall asleep again. She had many dreams and even nightmares. She felt as if she had not slept at night. During the day，she was mentally depressed，dizzy，tired，weak，irritable，emotional disordered，inattention and had poor memory.

Diagnosis：insomnia.

Drug treatment：3mg oral diazepam.

After taking medication，she could fall asleep very quickly in the evening. The medicine can help to reduce her dreams and sleep well.

Question：

1. Why can diazepam treat insomnia?

2. In addition to diazepam tablets，what other medications do you know for insomnia?

Discussion（问题讨论）

- What are the research contents of pharmacology?
- What is the purpose of pharmacodynamics research?
- What is the focus of pharmacokinetics research?
- What aspects do drugs mainly involve in the human body?

Reading Material（延伸阅读）

Principle of selecting medicine for hypertension
（高血压的选药原则）

There are many kinds of antihypertensive drugs commonly used in clinic.

Whatever drug is used, the aim of treatment is to control blood pressure within an ideal range to prevent or reduce target organ damage. The new guidelines emphasize that the choice of antihypertensive drugs should be based on the individual status of the treatment target, the role of drugs, metabolism, adverse reactions and drug interactions, with reference to the following points: (1) Whether the treatment target has cardiovascular risk factors; (2) Whether the treatment target has target organ damage and cardiovascular disease (especially coronary artery disease), the manifestations of atherosclerotic heart disease, nephropathy and diabetes mellitus; (3) Whether the subjects are complicated with other diseases affected by antihypertensive drugs; (4) Whether there is any possible interaction with the drugs used to treat the diseases; (5) Whether the drugs selected have evidence to reduce the incidence and mortality of cardiovascular diseases, and the supply and price situation of antihypertensive drugs and patient's ability to pay for treatment are also considered.

Lesson 6   Pharmacochemistry
第六课   药物化学

Situational Entry（情境导入）

The efficacy of drugs，especially natural medicines，is based on their active ingredients. A natural drug often contains many active ingredients，such as ephedrine，pseudoephedrine and other organic amine alkaloids in Chinese herbal medicine ephedra. For example，morphine in opium has analgesic effect，papaverine has antispasmodic effect，and codeine has antitussive effect. These three active ingredients in opium have different clinical uses. In order to obtain different bioactive ingredients，it is necessary to extract and separate the chemical components of drugs. In this lesson，we will learn about pharmaceutical chemistry.

Information about Pharmacochemistry（药物化学相关知识）

Pharmacochemistry studies the structure and activity of drugs on the basis of chemistry and biology. It involves the discovery，modification and optimization of main compounds，revealing the mechanism of action of drugs and biologically active substances at the molecular level，and studying the metabolic process of drugs and biologically active substances in the body.

Methods for extracting chemical components from natural medicines（天然药物化学成分的提取方法）

Natural medicines contain both active and inactive ingredients. To extract effective components is the most important step in the analysis of constituents present in natural medicine. Extraction refers to the process of dissolving all the chemical constituents in natural medicines as completely as possible from the tissues of medicinal materials. Extraction methods include solvent extraction，percolation，decoction，reflux，continuous reflux，ultrasonic extraction，steam distillation，sublimation and supercritical fluid method（shown as Fig. 6-1）.

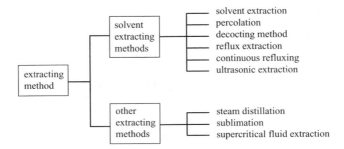

Fig. 6-1   Methods for extracting chemical components from natural medicines

Solvent extraction is a method for separating an active ingredient from medie inal materials based on its different solubility in two different immiscible liquids, usually water (polar) and an organic solvent (non-polar). This method is widely used in industry, and in laboratories for refining, isolating and purifying a variety of useful compounds. Percolation is a method to extract the ingredients from the medicinal materials by adding solvent from the upper part of the percolation tube. The decoction is the method to extract the essence from natural medicine by heating or boiling it. It is used for hard, woody substances (such as roots, bark, and stems) that have constituents that are water-soluble and non-volatile. Ultrasonic-assisted extraction is one of the most inexpensive, simple, rapid, and efficient green extraction techniques compared with conventional extraction and has been used to extract bioactive compounds from different materials due to its high reproducibility at shorter time, simplified manipulation. Steam distillation is a special type of distillation (a separation process) for temperature sensitive materials like natural aromatic compounds. Sublimation is the transition of a substance directly from the solid to the gas phase, without passing through the intermediate liquid phase. Supercritical fluid extraction (SFE) is the process of separating one component (the extractant) from another (the matrix) using supercritical fluids as the extracting solvent. Extraction is usually from a solid matrix, but can also be from liquids. SFE can be used as a sample preparation step for analytical purposes, or on a larger scale to strip unwanted material from a product.

Separation of chemical components from natural products (天然药物化学成分的分离方法)

The ingredients obtained from natural products after extracting are mixtures that contain many components. Further separation and purification is required to obtain the target component or monomers.

Common methods used for the separation target component from mixtures obtained from extracting include systematic solvent separation, two-phase solvent extraction, precipitation, crystallization and recrystallization, dialysis and fractionation. If extract from natural drugs contain some chemical substances with similar structure and properties, and general methods are not effective, we can choose the chromatography, such as alumina chromatography, silica gel chromatography and ion exchange chromatography, etc. (shown as Fig. 6-2).

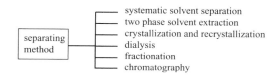

Fig. 6-2   Methods to separate chemical components from natural products

The systematic solvent separation is a method that can separate different components with different polarities by selecting different solvents according to the polarity order. It is one of the most important methods separating the active ingredients from natural products in the early years. At present, it is still widely used to separate unknown components from natural products. The two-phase solvent extraction is the method that can separate target component from a two-phase solvent system based on the different partition coefficients of the target components in the two-phase solvent. Precipitation refers to the method that can reduce the solubility of the target component and precipitate out of the solution by adding some reagents into the extraction solution, thus we can obtain effective components and remove impurities. Chromatography is a laboratory technique for the separation of a mixture. The mixture is dissolved in a fluid called the mobile phase, which carries it through a structure holding another material called the stationary phase. The various constituents of the mixture travel through the stationary phase at different speeds, causing them to separate.

Chemical constituents of natural medicines（天然药物的化学成分）

Natural medicine refers to animal medicine, plant medicine and mineral medicine with certain pharmacological activity proved by modern medicine system. Commonly active components include glycosides, alkaloid, quinones, flavonoids, terpenoids, volatile oil, etc.

Glycosides（糖类和苷类）

Glycosides are important natural products. They are derivatives of carbohydrates or saccharides, and widely distributed in plants. They have effects on cardiovascular system, respiratory system and digestive system. They are anti-bacterial, anti-inflammatory and anti-aging products. There are many effective components of carbohydrates and glycosides in nature, such as *Rehmannia glutinosa*. There are a lot of carbohydrates in *Rhizoma polygonatum*, Chinese yam, tremella fuciformis and astragalus membranaceus.

Alkaloid（生物碱）

Alkaloids are produced by a large variety of organisms including bacteria, fungi, plants, and animals. They can be purified from crude extracts of these organisms by acid-base extraction. Alkaloids have a wide range of pharmacological activities, including antimalarial（e. g. quinine）, antiasthma（e. g. ephedrine）, anticancer（e. g. homoharringtonine）.

Quinones（醌类）

Quinone compounds are natural compounds with unsaturated cyclodione structure or easily converted into this structure. They are mainly divided into benzoquinone, naphthoquinone, phenanthrenequinone and anthraquinone.

Flavonoids（黄酮类）

Flavonoids are natural compounds with the structure of 2-phenylchromone.

Terpenoids（萜类）

Terpenoids refer to hydrocarbons and their oxygenated derivatives that have multiple isoprene units in nature. These oxygen derivatives can be alcohols, aldehydes, ketones, carboxylic acids, esters, etc. Terpenoids are widely found in nature and are the main constituents of some plants such as essence, resin, pigment and so on. Rose oil, eucalyptus oil, turpentine contain a variety of terpenoids. In addition, some animal hormones, vitamins also belong to terpenoids.

Volatile oil（挥发油）

Volatile oils are a kind of volatile oily compounds with aromatic odor, which can be distilled with steam and is not miscible with water.

Vocabulary（课文词汇）

Pharmacochemistry 药物化学

modification 修正

optimization 优化

bioactive 生物活性

percolation 渗滤法

decoction 煎煮法

reflux 回流

ultrasonic extraction 超声波抽提

steam distillation 水蒸气蒸馏

sublimed method 升华法

supercritical fluid method 超临界流体法

solvent extraction 溶剂提取法

systematic solvent separation 系统溶剂分离法

two-phase solvent extraction 两相溶剂提取法

crystallization 结晶法

recrystallization 重结晶法

fractionation 分馏法

Summary（重点小结）

1. Extraction methods of chemical constituents of natural medicines include solvent extraction，percolation，decoction，reflux，continuous reflux，ultrasonic extraction，steam distillation，sublimation and supercritical fluid method.

2. Commonly used methods for the separation of chemical constituents of natural medicines include systematic solvent separation，two-phase solvent extraction，precipitation，crystallization and recrystallization，dialysis and fractionation.

3. Natural medicines have many active ingredients. Commonly active components include glycosides，alkaloid，quinones，flavonoids，terpenoids，volatile oil，etc.

4. Alkaloids are produced by a large variety of organisms including bacteria，

fungi，plants，and animals.

Quiz（课后检测）

Fill in the blanks.

1. _____ are natural compounds with the structure of 2-phenylchromone.

2. _____ refer to hydrocarbons and their oxygenated derivatives which are multiple of isoprene units in nature.

3. _____ are a kind of volatile oily compounds with aromatic odor，which can be distilled with steam and is not miscible with water.

4. _____ refers to animal medicine，plant medicine and mineral medicine with certain pharmacological activity proved by modern medicine system.

Discussion（问题讨论）

- What are the extraction methods of natural chemical components?
- What are the separation methods of natural chemical components?
- What are the chemical components of natural medicines?

Reading Material（延伸阅读）

New ideas on global natural drug research and development
（全球天然药物研发新思路）

Natural medicines are produced from natural material with pharmacological activities in nature，such as animals，plants and minerals. With the development of economy and the improvement of living level，the negative effects of chemicals on human health and environment have drawn great attention，and the demand for natural medicines in the international market is increasing. According to data released by China Industry Research Network，sales of natural medicines have reached 16 billion US dollars and are increasing at a rate of 10％ per year.

Because the natural medicine market is optimistic，many enterprises and scientists all over the world have devoted themselves to the development and research of natural medicine. He Yun，a senior research and development expert of new drugs，has been engaged in the research of bioactive natural products for 29 years since he started his PhD in 1988.

During September 8 to 10, the 2007 China Medical Innovation Summit Forum, participated by the Top 100 List of R&D strength of pharmaceutical enterprises, jointly sponsored by Pharmaceutical Intelligence Network and China Pharmacy magazine, held in Chongqing. Professor He Yun was invited to give a speech on the theme of "New Thoughts on Global Natural Drug Research and Development". He elaborated on the importance of natural product based drug research and development, and selected some cases to analyze the research process from natural products to marketed drugs, showing the role of synthetic chemistry, pharmaceutical chemistry and drug design in natural product drug research and development.

Lesson 7   Pharmaceutical Analysis
第七课   药物分析

Situational Entry（情境导入）

The connotation of drug quality includes three aspects：authenticity，purity and quality. The quality of drugs not only directly affects the effect of prevention and treatment of illness，but also closely related to the health and safety of consumers. Therefore，the quality of drugs must be strictly controlled. Drug analysis is to monitor the quality of drugs in drug research，production，circulation and clinical use. It plays a vital role in the quality control of drugs. In this lesson，we will learn the content of drug analysis together.

Information about pharmaceutical analysis（药物分析相关知识）

Substances used in medicine are to prevent diseases，cure diseases，diagnose diseases，improve physical fitness and enhance body resistance.

Pharmaceutical analysis is the study on composition，physicochemical properties，authenticity identification，purity test and determination of active ingredients of drugs and their preparations，which can ensure drug usage is safe，rational and effective.

Drug quality standard（药品质量标准）

Drug quality standards refer to the technical parameter and indicators that reflect the quality characteristics of drugs. These technical characteristics are clearly stipulated and technical documents are formed to formulate drug quality specifications and inspection methods. In order to ensure the quality of drugs，the requirements，indicators，limits and scopes of various inspection items have been formulated，which are called drug quality standards. Drug quality standard is a comprehensive expression of drug purity，composition，bioavailability，efficacy, toxicity, side effects, pyrogen, sterility and physical and chemical properties.

The pharmaceutical quality standard is divided into two types: statutory standard and enterprise standard. The statutory standards are also divided into national pharmacopoeia, industry standards and local standards. Pharmacopoeia shall be the standard for drug production. Drugs that fail to set standards and fail to meet statutory standards are not allowed to be produced, sold and used.

Pharmaceutical quality verification includes: accuracy, precision (including repeatability, intermediate precision and reproducibility), specificity, detection limit, quantitative limit, linearity, scope and durability. The content of validation is formulated according to specific methods.

The basic composition of Chinese Pharmacopoeia (《中国药典》的基本组成)

The Chinese Pharmacopoeia (CP) is the official general scientific and technical provisions for drug quality control and administration. The formulation of drug standards plays an important role in strengthening the supervision and management of drug quality, ensuring drug quality, drug safety and efficiency, and safeguarding people's health. Drug standard is an important part of modern drug production and quality management. It is the legal basis of the department of drug production, supply, use and supervision. The drug standard generally includes the following contents: legal name, source, characteristic, identification, purity examination, determination of content, category, dose, specification, storage, preparation, etc.

Basic procedures for pharmaceutical analysis and testing (药物分析与检验的基本程序)

The fundamental purpose of pharmaceutical analysis is to ensure the safety and effectiveness of drug use. Basic procedures for pharmaceutical analysis and testing is as following diagram (Fig. 7-1).

Sampling (抽样，取样)

Sampling is the first step in drug analysis. In order to ensure to be authentic and scientific of the drug analysis results, the scientificity of sampling should be considered.

Identification (鉴定)

The identification of drugs is based on the chemical structure and physicochemical

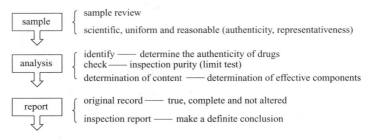

Fig. 7-1   Basic procedures for pharmaceutical analysis and testing

properties of the drugs，which can determine the authenticity of drugs and their preparations. The identification of drugs is not the analysis of the structure and composition of the unknown drugs，but the confirmation of known drugs.

Check（检验）

Drug testing includes testing for impurities and other items. Micro impurities are usually allowed for the production and storage of drugs without affecting their efficacy and safety. The maximum allowable amount of impurities is specified in the quality standards. As long as the impurities in the drug do not exceed this limit，the purity can be determined to meet the requirements. Therefore，the inspection of impurities can be referred to as a limit test or a purity test.

Content determination（含量测定）

Content determination of drugs is the determination of the main active ingredients in drugs. A chemical or physical chemical analysis is usually used to determine whether the drug content meets the quality standards.

Original records and inspection reports（原始记录和检验报告）

In the process of drug analysis and inspection，the inspection records must be filled out truthfully and shall not be changed at will. After all items are checked，a test report shall be issued based on the test results and a clear conclusion shall be drawn.

There are three situations that usually occur：①All indicators meet the requirements after the sample is fully inspected，which can be determined as qualified. ② After comprehensive inspection，some items do not meet the requirements but still can be used medicinally. ③All items or key items are below the standard or do not comply with the regulations after the sample is fully inspected，which can be identified as non-medicinally.

Drug quality management practice（药品质量管理规范）

Drug quality management practice is about the quality management of drug production in China，which includes GMP、GSP、GLP、GCP and GAP.

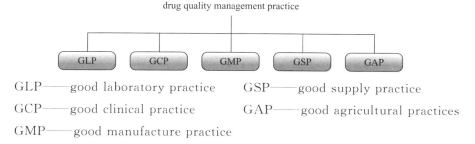

GLP——good laboratory practice   GSP——good supply practice

GCP——good clinical practice   GAP——good agricultural practices

GMP——good manufacture practice

Pharmaceutical analysis method（药物分析方法）

Pharmaceutical analysis method mainly includes chemical analysis and instrumental analysis methods. Chemical analysis methods include capacity analysis and gravimetric analysis method. Instrumental analysis methods include chromatographic analysis，spectral analysis，electrochemical analysis，NMR and MS techniques.

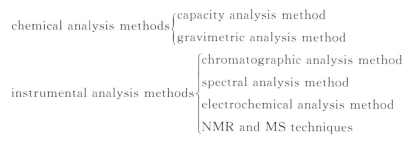

Vocabulary（课文词汇）

pharmaceutical analysis 药物分析

authenticity 真实性

parameters 参数

pharmacopoeia 药典

impurities 杂质

verification 检验

precision 准确性

inconsistent 不一致的

confirmation 确认

NMR：nuclear magnetic resonance 核磁共振

MS：mass spectrometer 质谱

Summary（重点小结）

1. Pharmaceutical analysis studies the composition，physicochemical properties，authenticity identification，purity test and determination of active ingredients of drugs and their preparations.

2. The Chinese Pharmacopoeia（CP）is the official general scientific and technical provision for drug quality control and administration.

3. Basic procedures for pharmaceutical analysis and testing include sampling，indentify，check，content determination，original records and inspection reports.

4. Chemical analysis methods include capacity analysis and gravimetric analysis method.

5. Instrumental analysis methods include chromatographic analysis，spectral analysis，electrochemical analysis，NMR and MS techniques.

Quiz（课后检测）

Ⅰ. **Fill in the blanks according to the information about Pharmaceutical analysis.**

1. Pharmaceutical analysis method mainly includes _____ and _____ .

2. _____ is the determination of the main active ingredients in drugs.

Ⅱ. **Translate the following English technological process into Chinese according to the knowledge of pharmaceutical analysis.**

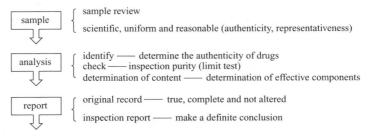

Discussion（问题讨论）

• What is the goal of setting up the drug quality standard?

- What is included in the Pharmacopoeia?
- What are the basic procedures for pharmaceutical analysis and testing?
- What are the methods of pharmaceutical analysis?

Reading Material（延伸阅读）

Effects of impurities on drug safety
（杂质对药物安全性的影响）

The relationship between drug impurities and drug safety is a complex one affected by many factors. Most of the impurities in drugs have potential biological activities，and some even interact with drugs to affect the efficacy and safety of drugs. Serious toxicity may occur. For example，the penicillin thiazole protein produced by beta-lactam ring has immunogenicity and is an exogenous allergen，and the macromolecule polymer produced by self-polymerization of the ring opening of -lactam ring during storage is an endogenous allergen. These are the reasons why lactam antibiotics are prone to allergic reactions. The common synthetic impurity，N-methyl-4-phenyl-1,2,3,6-tetrahydropyridine（MPTP），selectively destroys dopaminergic neurons in the substantia nigra and globus pallidus and induces symptoms similar to Parkinson's disease；degradation products in tetracycline cause Fanconi syndrome；and by-products of methotrexate produce febrile reactions. The optical isomerism of most drugs can affect the efficacy of drugs and even serious adverse reactions. For example，Thalidomide R-isomer and its two metabolites *in vivo* have strong embryotoxicity and teratogenicity.

Lesson 8   Pharmaceutical Dosage Forms
第八课　药物剂型

💡 Situational Entry（情境导入）

Any drug intended for the clinical treatment must be made into some forms suitable for medical and prophylactic applications, which is called dosage forms of drugs. In order to achieve the best therapeutic effect, the same drug can be processed into various dosage forms for clinical use according to the different route of administration. The different forms make patient use them easily. This can not only make sure the exact amount of drugs needed but also increases the stability of the drug. In some cases it also reduces the toxic side effects, and the drug is also easy to store, transport and carry, such as capsule, tablet, etc. (Fig. 8-1). We will give a brief introduction of pharmaceutical dosage forms on this topic.

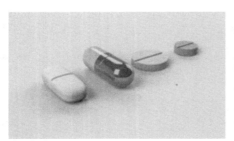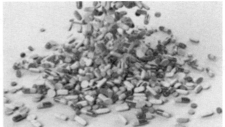

Fig. 8-1   Pharmaceutical dosage forms

Information about pharmaceutical dosage forms（药物剂型相关知识）

What is first-pass effect（首过效应）

First-pass effect is a phenomenon of drug metabolism whereby the concentration of a drug is greatly reduced before it reaches the systemic circulation. It is the fraction of the lost drug during the process of absorption，which is generally related to the liver and gut wall. A drug administered by mouth is absorbed from the gastrointestinal tract and transported via the portal vein to the liver，where it is metabolized. The pathway is：gut lumen（肠腔）→ gut wall（肠道壁）→ portal vein（门静脉）→ liver（肝脏）→systemic circulation（体循环）（Fig. 8-2）. As a result，in cases of some drugs，only a small proportion of the active drug reaches the systemic circulation and its intended target tissue.

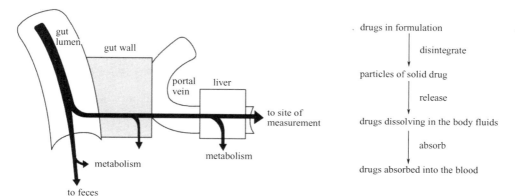

Fig. 8-2   The first-pass effect of the drugs

Bioavailability（生物利用度）

Bioavailability is the fraction of an administered dose of unchanged drug that reaches the systemic circulation，one of the principal pharmacokinetic properties of drugs. Bioavailability must be considered when calculating dosages for non-intravenous routes of administration.

Significance of dosage form design（药物剂型设计的重要性）

The dosage form can alter the drug effect. A good example is magnesium sulfate（硫酸镁）. Magnesium Sulfate powder can be used externally to reduce inflammation and swelling，help improve rough skin and help to repair muscle damage. Magnesium sulfate also can be used orally as a laxative to relieve occasional constipation.

The dosage form can alter the onset of action. For instance，the onset action of injection/sublingual tablet is quick，whereas the onset action of sustained release tablet is chronic.

The dosage form can alter the toxic and side effects. Aminophylline is used for the treatment of asthma. Oral administration can cause the toxic and side effects of rapid heartbeat. Suppositories can eliminate the toxic and side effects. Sustained and controlled release preparations can maintain stable drug concentration in blood，avoid peak-valley phenomenon of blood drug concentration，and reduce the toxic and side effects of drugs.

Some dosage forms have targeting effect，i. e.，targeted drug delivery system（靶向给药系统）. Also dosage forms can directly affect efficacy.

What are the pharmaceutical dosage forms?（什么是药物剂型？）

Pharmaceutical dosage form is the physical form of a chemical compound used as a drug or medication intended for administration or consumption（Fig. 8-3）. Dosage form can be a solid，liquid，semisolid and gaseous type shown below.

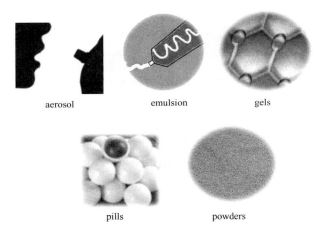

aerosol   emulsion   gels

pills   powders

Fig. 8-3   The different dosage form of the drugs

- Gaseous dosage forms：aerosol（气雾剂）.
- Liquid dosage forms：solution，emulsion（乳剂），syrup，injection，lotion（涂剂），suspension（混悬剂）.
- Semisolid dosage forms：gels（凝胶剂），creams（乳膏），ointments（软膏剂），pastes（糊剂）.
- Solid dosage forms：tablet，capsule，pills（丸剂），powders（散剂）.

Effervescent tablet（泡腾片）

Effervescent tablets are uncoated tablets that generally contain acid substances and carbonates or bicarbonates that react rapidly in the presence of water by releasing carbon dioxide. They are intended to be dissolved or dispersed in water before use.

Buccal tablet（口含片）

The buccal tablet is usually a small，flat tablet intended to be inserted in the buccal pouch（颊囊），where the active ingredient is absorbed directly through the oral mucosa. This kind of tablet dissolves or erodes slowly.

Sublingual tablet（舌下片）

Usually，a small，flat tablet intended to be inserted beneath the tongue，where the active ingredient is absorbed directly through the oral mucosa and into blood. This kind of tablet dissolves very promptly.

Nitroglycerin sublingual tablet is a type of vasodilator. It relaxes blood vessels，increasing the blood and oxygen supply to your heart. This medicine is used to relieve chest pain caused by angina.

Enteric coated tablet（肠溶片）

Enteric coated tablet is an oral dosage form. The tablet is coated with a material to prevent or minimize dissolution in the stomach but allow dissolution in the small intestine. This type of formulation either protects the stomach from a potentially irritating drug（e. g.，aspirin）or protects the drug（e. g.，erythromycin）from partial degradation in the acidic environment of the stomach.

Hard capsule（硬胶囊）

The shell of hard gelatin capsules basically consists of gelatin，plasticizers（增塑剂）and water. The plasticizers used are glycerin（甘油），sorbitol（山梨醇），etc.

Soft capsule（软胶囊）

The composition of soft gelatin capsule shells is similar to the hard gelatin capsules except that a larger proportion of plasticizer is incorporated to make them soft and elastic.

Suspension（混悬剂）

The suspension is a dispersion containing finely divided insoluble material suspended in a liquid medium. The solid particles are dispersed throughout the

medium through mechanical agitation，with the use of certain suspending agents
（助悬剂）.

Emulsions（乳剂）

Emulsions are biphasic systems consisting of two immiscible liquids，one of which（the dispersed phase，分散相）is finely subdivided and uniformly dispersed as droplets throughout the other phase（the continuous phase，连续相）. These immiscible liquids are made miscible by adding a third substance known as emulsifying agent（乳化剂）. They stabilize the system by forming a thin film around the globules of the dispersed phase.

Ointment（油膏）

An ointment is a homogeneous，viscous，semi-solid preparation that is intended for external application to the skin or mucous membranes. Ointments are used on a variety of body surfaces. These include the skin and the mucous membranes of the eye.

Transdermal patch（透皮贴剂）

A transdermal patch is a medicated adhesive patch that is placed on the skin to deliver a specific dose of medication through the skin and into the bloodstream.

Aerosol（气雾剂）

Aerosol is packaged under pressure and contains therapeutically active ingredients that are released upon activation of an appropriate valve system. The basic components of an aerosol system are listed below.

- pressurizable container（耐压容器）
- nozzle（喷嘴）
- metering valve（定量阀）
- mixtures of liquid drug and liquefied gas（液化气体）
- dip tube（汲取管）

Vocabulary（课文词汇）

pharmaceutics 制剂，药剂学

chemical entity 化学品

dosage form 剂型

first-pass effect 首过效应

absorption 吸收

suspension 混悬剂

tablet 片剂

intravenous 静脉注射

capsule 胶囊

effervescent tablet 泡腾片

sublingual 舌下的

buccal tablet 口含片

ointment 软膏剂

transdermal patch 透皮贴剂

aerosol 气雾剂

emulsion 乳剂

enteric coated tablet 肠溶剂

Summary（重点小结）

1. First-pass effect is a phenomenon of drug metabolism whereby the concentration of a drug is greatly reduced before it reaches the systemic circulation.

2. Effervescent tablets are uncoated tablets that generally contain acid substances and carbonates or bicarbonates that react rapidly in the presence of water by releasing carbon dioxide.

3. The suspension is a dispersion containing finely divided insoluble material suspended in a liquid medium.

4. A transdermal patch is a medicated adhesive patch that is placed on the skin to deliver a specific dose of medication through the skin and into the bloodstream.

5. The shell of hard gelatin capsules basically consists of gelatin、plasticizers（增塑剂）and water. The plasticizers used are glycerin（甘油）, sorbitol（山梨醇）, etc.

6. An ointment is a homogeneous、viscous、semi-solid preparation that is intended for external application to the skin or mucous membranes.

Quiz（课后检测）

Ⅰ. **Fill in the blanks according to the information about pharmaceutical dosage forms.**

1. _____ is usually a small，flat tablet intended to be inserted in the buccal pouch.

2. _____ is used to relieve chest pain caused by angina.

3. _____ are biphasic systems consisting of two immiscible liquids，one of which（the dispersed phase）is finely subdivided and uniformly dispersed as droplets throughout the other phase（the continuous phase）.

4. _____ is the physical form of a dose of a chemical compound used as a drug or medication intended for administration or consumption.

Ⅱ. **Please place the drugs in the pictures below into the right category.**

(   ) belong to the tablet.

(   ) belong to the capsule.

(   ) belong to the injection.

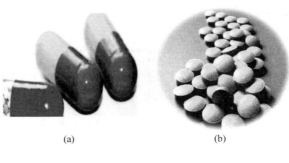

(a)   (b)

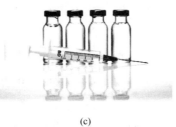

(c)

Discussion（问题讨论）

- Why do you choose the effervescent tablet?

- What is the bioavailability of drugs?
- What is the difference between the soft capsule and hard capsule?
- What is the dosage form of the drugs?

Reading Material（延伸阅读）

Pharmacy English dialogue
（日常药房用语）

Patient：I have a terrible cold. Apart from that，I have a headache. Can you suggest something I can take to relieve the pain?

Pharmacist：Don't you have a prescription?

Patient：No，I haven't gone to see a doctor.

Pharmacist：Are you allergic to any type of medication?

Patient：I don't know exactly. I think that I can take most drugs.

Pharmacist（picks up a small box）：I recommend this brand for quick relief.

Patient：Will this really help?

Pharmacist：According to the label，yes. But if that doesn't help，then drink a cup of hot tea along with some honey. There's no miracle drug to cure a common cold.

Patient：Which are the best headache tablets?

Pharmacist：We have a number of them. They are all very good.

Patient：Can you sell me penicillin?

Pharmacist：Sorry，sir. I can not sell it，you must first get a doctor's certificate or prescription.

Patient：Well，then. Give me some boric acid.

Pharmacist：All right. This is a common medicine.

Patient：Do you have any cough syrup and lozenges?

Pharmacist：Of course.

Patient：That's great.

Pharmacist：Here you are. The instructions on it tell you how to take it. Make sure you read them carefully.

Patient：Thank you for reminding me.

Unit 3
Medicine Sale and Management
第三单元　药品销售和管理

Lesson 9　Medicines and Pharmacists
第九课　药品和药剂师

Situational Entry（情境导入）

It happens you encounter a foreigner to buy drugs. He has a sore throat and knows Chinese little (Fig. 9-1). You may often see some imported drugs without instructions in Chinese in the drugstore (Fig. 9-2). Therefore we have to learn necessary professional pharmacy English so that we can work better in the future. Because the basic job of a pharmacist is to guide patients to purchase medication，we will give a brief introduction of drugs and pharmacists on this topic.

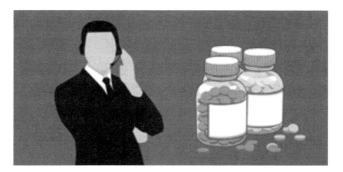

Fig. 9-1　The case of buying the drugs

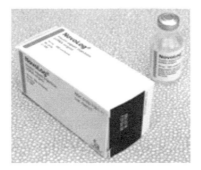

Fig. 9-2　Imported drugs

What are medicines?（什么是药品？）

Medicines refer to those substances used for the prevention，treatment，and diagnosis of human diseases，and for the intentional regulation of human physiological functions. To instruct how to use drugs，usage and dosage have been established. They include herbal medicines and their preparations，prepared slice of herbal medicines，chemical medicines and their preparations，antibiotics，biochemical medicines，radioactive pharmaceuticals，sera and vaccines，blood products，diagnostic aids etc. （Fig. 9-3）.

What is a pharmacist?（什么是药剂师？）

Pharmacists are health professionals who，in addition to dispensing prescription medication to patients，also provide information about the drugs their doctors have ordered for them. They explain doctors' instructions to patients so

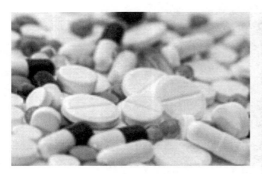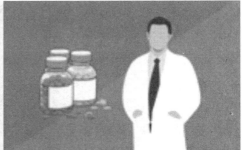

Fig. 9-3   Drugs and pharmacist

that these individuals can use these medications safely and effectively (Fig. 9-3).

What is the working content of a pharmacist? (药剂师的工作内容是什么?)

Pharmacists distribute drugs prescribed by physicians and other health practitioners and provide information to patients about medications and their usage. They advise physicians and other health practitioners on the selection，dosages，interactions，and side effects of medications. Pharmacists also monitor the health and progress of patients in response to drug therapy to ensure the safe and effective use of medication. Pharmacists must understand the use，clinical effects，and composition of drugs，including their chemical，biological，and physical properties. Most pharmacists work in a community setting，such as a retail drugstore，or in a healthcare facility，such as a hospital，nursing home，mental health institution，or neighborhood health clinic.

Working Conditions (工作条件)

Pharmacists work in clean，well-lighted，and well-ventilated areas. Many pharmacists spend most of their workday on their feet. When working with sterile or dangerous pharmaceutical products，pharmacists wear gloves and masks and work with other special protective equipment.

Training，other qualifications and promotions (培训、其他资格和晋升)

Here we only introduce some facts in USA. A license to practice pharmacy is required in all states，the District of Columbia，and all U. S. territories. To obtain a license，the prospective pharmacist must graduate from a college of pharmacy that is accredited by the Accreditation Council for Pharmacy Education (ACPE) and passes an examination. All states require the North American Pharmacist Licensure Exam (NAPLEX), which tests pharmacy skills and knowledge. And 43 states and the District of Columbia require the Multistate Pharmacy Jurisprudence Exam (MPJE), which tests pharmacy law. Both exams are administered by the National Association of Boards of Pharmacy. Pharmacists in other states that do not require the MJPE must pass a state-specific exam that is similar to the MJPE. In addition to the NAPLEX and MPJE, some states require additional exams unique to their state. All states except California currently grant a license without extensive reexamination to qualified pharmacists who already are licensed by another state. In Florida, reexamination is not required if a pharmacist has passed the NAPLEX and MPJE within 12 years of his or her application for a license transfer. Many pharmacists are licensed to practice in more than one state. Most states require continuing education for license renewal. Prospective pharmacists should have scientific aptitude, good communication skills, and a desire to help others. They also must be conscientious and pay close attention to detail, because the decisions they make affect human lives.

Applications（应用实例）

The pharmacists in the United States share high social status as doctors and lawyers. They are responsible for rechecking the prescriptions prescribed by doctors, monitoring and guiding non-prescription drugs, consulting and coaching the customers. In 2009, licensed pharmacists were named the ten largest female gold profession in the United States. They help consumers with prescriptions and give instructions on the safe use of medications (Fig. 9-4).

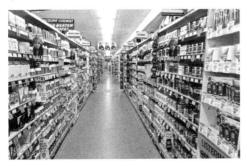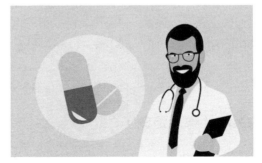

Fig. 9-4 Prescriptions and instructions by the pharmacist

Vocabulary（课文词汇）

pharmacist 药剂师

physician 医师

side effect 副作用

medication 药物

ventilated 通风的

license 执照

accredited 认证过的

prospective 前景

territory 地区，领土

qualification 任职资格

district 地区

institution 学院，研究机构

retail 零售，零售的

dosages 剂量

Summary（重点小结）

1. Drugs refer to those substances used for the prevention，treatment and diagnosis of human diseases，and for the intentional regulation of human physiological functions.

2. Pharmacists are health professionals who，in addition to dispensing prescription medication to patients，also provide information about the drugs their doctors have ordered for them.

3. Pharmacists work in clean，well-lighted，and well-ventilated areas.

4. To obtain a license，the prospective pharmacist must graduate from a college of pharmacy that is accredited by the Accreditation Council for Pharmacy Education（ACPE）and passes an examination.

5. Pharmacists distribute drugs prescribed by physicians and other health practitioners and provide information to patients about medications and their usage.

Quiz（课后检测）

Ⅰ. **Fill in the blanks according to the information about pharmacists.**

1. _____ explain doctors' instructions to patients so that these individuals can

use these medications safely and effectively.

2. _____ include herbal drugs and their preparations.

3. They advise physicians and other health practitioners on the _____, _____ interactions, and _____ of medications.

4. Prospective _____ should have scientific aptitude, good communication skills, and a desire to help others.

II. It is illegal for pharmacists to sell prescription-only drugs without a prescription unless it is a medical emergency. What do you think?

Discussion (问题讨论)

- What are medicines?
- What is a pharmacist?
- What is the difference between drugs and medicine?
- What is the working condition of pharmacists?

Reading Material (延伸阅读)

Pharmacists employment
(药剂师就业)

In December 2016, according to the survey by Gallup, a famous American public opinion survey company, 70% of American citizens expressed full trust in pharmacists, the second most trusted by the American people, second only to the number one, nurse.

There were 274,900 registered pharmacists in the United States, according to statistics by the end of 2016, and the number is expected to increase by 25% in 2020. More than 65% of the pharmacists are employed by retail pharmacies. In addition, 22% of pharmacists work in hospitals, while the rest are distributed in mail order pharmacies and online pharmacies. Pharm. D. is the first professional degree of a pharmacist. It takes 4 years to complete the doctor of pharmacy. The first 3 years are compulsory basic courses. Besides pharmacy, there are medicine, ethics, patient communication and how to cooperate with the doctor courses. In the 2nd and 3rd years, students should choose the direction of their work, and choose related courses such as drug treatment, biostatistics, health management, or clinical specialties. The 4th year is for completing clinical training for pharmacists, including the diagnosis and guidance of patients in hospitals and pharmacists. Each rotation lasts for 4~6 weeks, and most students need to complete 7~10 turns to graduate. After completing the Pharm. D. , the pharmacist will also have to pass the pharmacist's examination NAPLEX, MPJE or FPGEC.

Comparing with Americans, it's so easy to be a licensed pharmacist in China.

Lesson 10   Classification of the Medicines
第十课   药品的分类

Situational Entry（情境导入）

We often see various drug labels in the pharmacy as shown in the picture below（Fig. 10-1）. You may have the experience that you cannot purchase some antibiotics without a doctor's prescription. But some medicines can be bought in the drugstore without a doctor's prescription. We will give a brief introduction of classification of drugs on this topic.

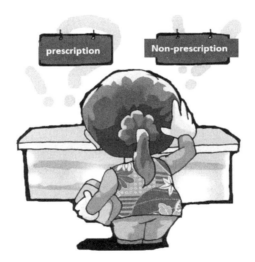

Fig. 10-1   Types of drug labels in the pharmacy

Classification management of drugs（药品分类管理）

Classification management of drugs is a common international management method. Based on the principles of safety and effectiveness of drugs，drugs are classified into prescription drugs and non-prescription drugs according to their varieties，specifications，indications，dosages and delivery routes. Through the classification management of drugs，on the one hand，it can strengthen the supervision and management of prescription drugs to prevent consumers from abusing drugs and endangering their health due to improper self-behavior; on the other hand, it can guide consumers to conduct self-care scientifically and reasonably by standardizing the management of over-the-counter drugs.

What is the prescription medicines (Rx)? (什么是处方药?)

Rx is a common abbreviation for medical prescriptions. The "R" in "Rx" stands for the Latin word recipe, meaning "take". Prescription medicines can be purchased and used with a doctor's prescription. Ninety percent antibiotics are prescription medicines, such as penicillin, erythromycin, cephalexin, etc. (Fig. 10-2).

What are the non-prescription medicines (OTC)? (什么是非处方药?)

Non-prescription medicine is over the counter (OTC) medicine. According to the level of its security, it can be divided into class Jia and class Yi. The red sign on OTC package is called class Jia, the green logo is called class Yi (Fig. 10-2, and see colored picture).

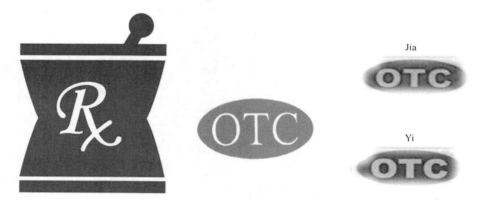

Fig. 10-2   The logo of the prescription and non-prescription

The prescription drug——antibiotics (处方药——抗生素)

Antibiotics, sometimes known as antibacterial drugs, are used to treat infections caused by bacteria. There are tiny organisms, too small to see with naked eyes, which sometimes cause illness in human. Well-known illnesses caused by bacteria include tuberculosis, salmonella, syphilis and some forms of meningitis. Many types of bacteria do not cause illness and live harmlessly on and in the human body. Our immune systems, with their antibodies and special white blood cells, can usually kill harmful bacteria before they multiply enough to cause symptoms. Even when symptoms do occur, the body can often fight off the infection. However, sometimes the body is overwhelmed by a bacterial infection and needs help to get rid of it. This is where antibiotics come in. An antibiotic is a substance produced by a microorganism capable of destroying or inhibiting the growth of other microorganisms. The production of such substances is one of the means used by microorganisms to compete with other microorganisms for survival in their highly competitive environment. The very first antibiotic was penicillin and along with a family of related antibiotics (such as ampicillin, amoxicillin and benzylpenicillin). It is still widely used to treat many common infections. Now there are several other different kinds of antibiotics. All of them are only available from prescription.

How do antibiotics work? (抗生素是如何发挥作用的?)

Some antibiotics, such as penicillin (discovered by English bacteriologist Alexander Fleming in 1928), are "bactericidal", meaning that they work by killing bacteria. They do this by interfering with the formation of the cell walls or cell contents of the bacteria. Other antibiotics are "bacteriostatic", meaning that they work by stopping bacteria multiplying.

What are antibiotics for? (抗生素的作用是什么?)

Antibiotics are usually used to treat infections caused by bacteria. They do not work against other organisms such as viruses or fungi. It's important to bear this in mind if you think you have some sort of infection, because many common illnesses, particularly of the upper respiratory tract such as the common cold and sore throats, are usually caused by viruses. Overuse of antibiotics can lead to bacteria becoming resistant to them, it's important to only take them when necessary. Some antibiotics can be used to treat a wide range of infections and are known as "broad-spectrum" antibiotics. Others are only effective against a few types of bacteria and are called "narrow-spectrum" antibiotics. Some antibiotics work against aerobic bacteria that are organisms that need oxygen to live. While others work against anaerobic bacteria, which are organisms that don't need oxygen. Sometimes antibiotics are given to prevent an infection occurring, for example，before certain operations. This is known as the prophylactic use of antibiotics and is common before orthopedic and bowel surgery.

Side effects of antibiotics（抗生素的副作用）

The most common side effects of antibiotic drugs are diarrhea，feeling sick and being sick. Fungal infections of the mouth，digestive tract and vagina can also occur with antibiotics because they destroy the protective "good" bacteria in the body（which help prevent overgrowth of any bad organism），as well as the "bad" ones，responsible for the infection being treated.

Use antibiotics with care（谨慎使用抗生素）

You should use an antibiotic with care if you have reduced liver or kidney function. You should avoid using any antibiotic to which you previously had an allergic reaction. Tell your doctor or pharmacist if you are pregnant or breast-feeding before taking any antibiotic. Interactions can occur with other medicines. Do not take any other medicines or herbal remedies with an antibiotic，including those you have bought without a prescription，before talking to your doctor or pharmacist. Certain antibiotics（e. g. penicillin，cephalosporin）can reduce the effectiveness of oral contraceptives. If you have diarrhea or vomiting while taking an antibiotic，the absorption of the pill can be disrupted. In either case，you should take additional precautions while you are taking the antibiotic. There are a number of interactions between antibiotics and other medicines，so it's important to tell your doctor or pharmacist the medicine you are taking.

How to use an antibiotic correctly?（如何正确使用抗生素?）

Antibiotics are usually taken orally but can also be given by injection，or applied to the affected part of the body such as the skin，eyes or ears. The drugs begin to tackle most infection within a few hours. It is vital to take the whole course of treatment to prevent recurrence of the infection. Sometimes bacteria become "resistant" to an antibiotic you have been taking，meaning that the drug will no longer work. Resistance tends to occur when the bacterial infection responsible for the symptoms is not completely cured，even if the symptoms have cleared up. Some of the residual bacteria，having been exposed to，but not killed by the antibiotic are more likely to grow into an infection that can survive that particular antibiotic. This explains why finishing the course of antibiotics， even if you feel better，is important. Certain antibiotics should not be taken with certain foods and drinks. Some antibiotics are best taken when there is no food in your stomach，usually an hour before meals or two hours after. Make sure you follow the instructions on the dispensing label. Do not drink alcohol if you are taking antibiotics.

Applications（应用实例）

By the end of the World War Ⅱ（WWⅡ），enough penicillin was produced to treat seven million patients every year. During World War Ⅰ（WWⅠ），the death rate from pneumonia in the american army totaled 18%. In WWⅡ，it fell to less than 1%. The discovery of penicillin makes people find a strong medicine to fight disease-causing bacteria. It ended the era of no treatment for infections and rose the climax to research new antibiotics（Fig. 10-3，and see colored picture）.

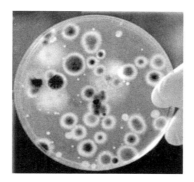

Fig. 10-3   The discovery of penicillin

Vocabulary（课文词汇）

    prescription 处方药
    OTC 非处方药
    erythromycin 红霉素
    penicillin 盘尼西林
    cephalexin 头孢氨苄
    non-prescription 非处方药
    antibacterial 抗细菌
    syphilis 梅毒
    amoxicillin 阿莫西林
    cephalosporin 头孢菌素
    dispense 分配

contraceptive 避孕药

breastfeeding 母乳喂养

spectrum 光谱

Summary（重点小结）

1. Prescription drugs can be purchased and used with a doctor's prescription. Ninety percent antibiotics are prescription drugs.

2. Non-prescription drug is over the counter drug.

3. Antibiotics，sometimes known as antibacterial drugs，are drugs used to treat infections caused by bacteria.

4. Certain antibiotics (e. g. penicillin，cephalosporin) can reduce the effectiveness of oral contraceptives.

5. Antibiotics are usually taken orally but can also be given by injection，or applied to the affected part of the body such as the skin，eyes or ears.

Quiz（课后检测）

Ⅰ. **Fill in the blanks according to the information about drugs.**

1. _____ do this by interfering with the formation of the cell walls or cell contents of the bacteria.

2. _____ is usually used to treat infections caused by bacteria.

3. According to the level of its security，it can be divided into _____ and _____ .

4. Ninety percent antibiotics are _____ drugs，such as penicillin，erythromycin，cephalexin，etc.

Ⅱ. **Which statement of the following pictures〔(a)、(b)〕is right? Give explanation.**

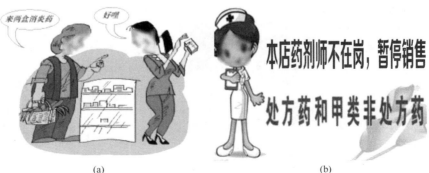

(a)   (b)

Discussion（问题讨论）

- Why do you choose the antibiotics?
- What is the principle of antibiotics' anti-infection?
- What is the difference between Rx and OTC?
- What is the side effect of antibiotic medicines?
- How to use an antibiotic correctly?
- What is the purpose of using antibiotics?

Reading Material（延伸阅读）

Antibiotic resistance could bring "the end of modern medicine"
（抗生素耐药性可能带来"现代医学的终结"）

As bacteria evolve to evade antibiotics, common infections could become deadly, according to Dr. Margaret Chan, Director-General of the World Health Organization. Speaking at a conference in Copenhagen, Chan said antibiotic resistance could bring "the end of modern medicine as we know it." "We are losing our first-line antimicrobials", she said in her keynote address at the conference on combating antimicrobial resistance. "Replacement treatments are more costly, more toxic, need much longer durations of treatment, and may require treatment in intensive care units." Chan said hospitals have become "hotbeds for highly-resistant pathogens" like methicillin-resistant *Staphylococcus aureus*, "increasing the risk that hospitalization kills instead of cures." Indeed, diseases that were once curable, such as tuberculosis, are becoming harder and more expensive to treat. Chan said treatment of multidrug resistant tuberculosis was "extremely complicated, typically requiring two years of medication with toxic and expensive medicines, some of which are in constant short supply. Even with the best of care, only slightly more than 50 percent of these patients will be cured." Antibiotic-resistant strains of *Salmonella*, *E. coli*, and gonorrhea have also been discovered. "Some experts say we are moving back to the pre-antibiotic era. No. This will be a post-antibiotic era. In terms of new replacement antibiotics, the pipeline is virtually dry," said Chan. "A post-antibiotic era means, in effect, an end to modern medicine as we know it. Things as common as strep throat or a child's scratched knee could once again kill."

The dearth of effective antibiotics could also make surgical procedures and certain cancer treatments risky or even impossible, Chan said. "Some sophisticated interventions, like hip replacements, organ transplants, cancer chemotherapy and care of preterm infants, would become far more difficult or even too dangerous to undertake," she said. The development of new antibiotics now could help stave off catastrophe later. But few drug makers are willing to invest in drugs designed for short-term use. "It's simply not profitable for them," said Dr. William Schaffner, chairman of preventive medicine at Vanderbilt University Medical Center in Nashville. "If you create a new drug to lower cholesterol, people will be taking that drug every day for the rest of their lives. But you only take antibiotics for a week or maybe 10 days." Schaffner likened the dilemma to Ford releasing a car that could only be driven if every other vehicle wasn't working. "While we try to encourage the pharmaceutical industry to create new antibiotics, we have to be very prudent in their use," he said. But there are ways to limit the potential for bacteria to develop antibiotic resistance: use antibiotics appropriately and only when needed; follow treatment correctly, and restrict the use of antibiotics in food production to therapeutic purposes. "At a time of multiple calamities in the world, we cannot allow the loss of essential antimicrobials, essential cures for many millions of people, to become the next global crisis," said Chan.

Lesson 11   Drug Regulation
第十一课　药物管制

Situational Entry（情境导入）

With the development of national economy，the progress of science and technology，especially the improvement of people's living standards，drug safety has drawn and will continue to draw the attention of the whole society. In each stage of social development，various problems have different characteristics. However，because drug safety is directly related to people's health and their right to survival，it is extremely likely to cause social shock if there are problems with it. As a result，drug safety has always been a major concern of the government at all levels. The pharmaceutical industry is one of the most tightly regulated areas by the government. We will give a brief introduction of drug regulation on this topic.

Information about drug regulation（药物管制相关知识）

Drug regulation is the application of government control in the pharmaceutical industry，and it is the administrative management and supervision of a series of links from drug research and development to use by government regulatory agencies. It aims at ensuring consumers to obtain more information about drugs and medical care services from the system，thus reducing transaction costs and health risks. Controlled drugs mainly include psychotropic drugs，narcotic drugs，ephedrine containing preparations，codeine containing preparations and diphenoxylate containing preparations.

Why should drugs be regulated?（为什么要进行药品管制?）

Drugs are not ordinary merchandise. Consumers are usually not in a position to make decisions about when to use drugs，which drugs to use，how to use them and to weigh potential benefits against risks，as no medicine is completely safe. Professional advises from either prescribers or dispensers are needed in making these decisions. However, even healthcare professionals (medical doctors, pharmacists) nowadays are not in capacity to take informed decisions about all aspects of medicines without special training and access to necessary information. The use of ineffective, poor quality, harmful medicines can result in therapeutic failure, exacerbation of disease, resistance to medicines, and sometimes death. It also undermines confidence in health systems, health professionals, pharmaceutical manufacturers and distributors. Money spent on ineffective, unsafe and poor quality medicines is wasted, whether by patients/consumers or insurance companies/governments. Government is responsible for protecting their citizens. Thus, governments need to establish strong national regulatory authorities (NRAs) to ensure that the manufacture, trade and use of medicines are regulated effectively. In broad terms, the mission of NRAs is to protect and promote public health. Medicine regulation demands the application of sound scientific (including but not limited to medical, pharmaceutical, biological and chemical) knowledge and specific technical skills, and operates within a legal framework.

The role of China's drug supervising agencies (中国药品监督管理机构的作用)

The government eventually control directly almost all privately owned pharmaceutical enterprises in China. In order to operate and regulate these enterprises, two administrative systems were established by the goverment after 1949. One was comprised by the competent departments for state-owned pharmaceutical enterprises. Another system was the drug supervising, which was for drug quality control.

The competent departments were a series of administrative bodies assigned to represent the government to perform the function of ownership. The head of state-owned pharmaceutical enterprises was responsible for management at the operational level, but decision-making and programming were performed by the competent departments of the government. In order to supervise the quality of the work of the competent departments, China established a drug supervising system. This system was a branch of the Ministry of health. The employees were primarily responsible for the management of state-owned hospitals as well as quality control over pharmaceutical products. They are responsible for the work to make regulations, set up national drug standards, approve grants and issue licenses.

What is registration of drugs?（什么是药品注册？）

Registration of drugs，also known as product licensing or marketing authorization，is an essential element of drug regulation. All drugs that are marketed，distributed and used in the country should be registered by the national competent regulatory authority. Only the inspection of manufacturing plants and laboratory quality control analysis certainly do not guarantee product quality and safety. Drug regulation should therefore include the scientific evaluation of products before registration，to ensure that all marketed pharmaceutical products meet the criteria of safety，efficacy and quality. Although these criteria are applicable to all medicines including biological products（vaccines，blood products，monoclonal antibodies，cell and tissue therapies）and herbal medicines（also other traditional and complementary medicines），there are substantial differences in the regulatory requirements for some groups of medicines.

Vocabulary（课文词汇）

drug regulation 药物管制

pharmaceutical industry 制药工业

supervision 监督；管理

codeine 可待因

psychotropic （药物）作用于精神的

competent department 主管部门

pharmaceutical enterprise 医药企业

narcotic 麻醉的；催眠的；吸毒成瘾的

approve 批准、同意

grant 授予、赋予

monoclonal antibody 单克隆抗体

substantial 大量的；结实的，重大的

implement 实施

Summary（重点小结）

1. Governments need to establish strong national regulatory authorities（NRAs）

to ensure that the manufacture，trade and use of medicines are regulated effectively.

2. The managers of state-owned pharmaceutical enterprises were responsible for management at the operational level，but decision-making and planning were performed by the competent departments of the government.

3. Registration of drugs，also known as product licensing or marketing authorization，is an essential element of drug regulation.

4. Drug regulation should therefore include the scientific evaluation of products before registration，to ensure that all marketed pharmaceutical products meet the criteria of safety，efficacy and quality.

Quiz（课后检测）

Fill in the blanks.

1. _____ from either prescribers or dispensers are needed in making these decisions.

2. _____ is the application of government control in the pharmaceutical industry.

3. The use of ineffective，poor quality，harmful medicines can _____ therapeutic failure，exacerbation of disease，resistance to medicines，and sometimes death.

4. _____ of drugs，also known as product licensing or marketing authorization，is an essential element of drug regulation.

Discussion（问题讨论）

- Why should drugs be regulated?
- What is the role of China's drug supervising agencies?
- What is registration of drugs?

Reading Material（延伸阅读）

Thirty-two drugs are included in the regulation
（32 种药品纳入管制）

The State Drug Control Office announced on August 29，2018 that in accordance with the regulations on the administration of narcotic drugs and psychotropic substances and the regulations on the listing and control of non-pharmaceutical narcotic drugs and psychotropic substances, the ministry of public security, the National Health Commission and the State Drug Administration have decided to list 32 substances, such as 4-chloroethylcarbazedone, as non-pharmaceutical narcotic drugs. And the catalogue of supplementary substances for psychotropic substances control came into effect on September 1st.

Neopsychological active substances, also known as "mastermind drugs" or "laboratory drugs", are drug analogues modified by lawbreakers in order to avoid being caught. They have the effects of excitement, similar to those of drug controlled. Deng Ming, deputy director of the state anti-drug office and deputy director of the anti-drug bureau of the ministry of public security, addressed that this third-generation drug, which has been spreading around the world since its emergence in 2009, is the most intractable and prominent problem in the field of international drug control in recent years.

Doctor Hua Zhendong of laboratory of national drug control office introduced that those 32 kinds of pure substance included in the list of controlled could rarely be accessed by ordinary people. However, the investigation discovered that various forms of drugs containing these pure substances had been illegally used in entertainment places.

The investigation of the national narcotics control office has found that, with the development and changes of the international drug situation, new features of psychoactive substances are constantly emerging. First, non-regulated substances with new structures are constantly emerging. Once a certain variety included under the control, criminals will develop new non-regulated substances in a short period of time. Second, the trading methods are diversified and more covert, such as overseas criminals network and selling via Skype, underground banks, Bitcoin and other new ways. Third, cases of abuse of new psychoactive substances began to increase in China. In addition to ketamine, other new psychoactive substances such as synthetic cannabinoids and methylcarasidone have been found in many places of entertainment, in Guangdong, Zhejiang, Yunnan, Xinjiang and Inner Mongolia.

Since 2001, the control of new psychoactive substances has been implemented in China, and the control has been gradually strengthened. By September 2018, 170 new psychoactive substances have been listed in China, including 25 new psychoactive substances listed as fentanyl, exceeding the international control level.

Lesson 12 Insert
第十二课 药品说明书

🔖 Situational Entry（情境导入）

We need to take medication when we are sick. Medicine insert is the integrated information of the medicines. The usage, the dosage and other characteristics of medicines should all be included in the medicine insert. This is the basis that pharmacists give the guidance of medication to the patients. There is a case that an old lady misunderstood the medicine instructions and was sent to emergency room after taking the medicine. Therefore, it is very important to read correctly the medicine inserts (Fig. 12-1).

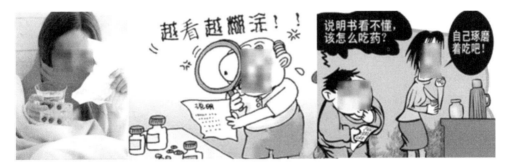

Fig. 12-1 The problem of reading the drug instructions

According to the FDA regulation, items in medicine insert include drug name, description, pharmacological actions, indication, contraindication, precaution, side effects, dosage and administration, packing, expiration date, manufacture date. According to the drug law, there are at least three names for a chemical drug. They are trade name, generic name, and chemical name. The most common trade name is protected by law. Register means that the product has been approved by the relevant departments of the country, and it has obtained the registered trademark for this special purpose. Below is an example of a medicine insert of trimetazidine dihydrochloride tablets.

Insert of Trimetazidine Dihydrochloride

[Drug names]

　　Generic name: Trimetazidinedihydrochloride tablets

　　English name: Trimetazidine Dihydrochloride Tablets

　　Chinese Pinyin: Yan Suan Qu Mei Ta Qin Pian

[Ingredients]

　　Chemical name: Trimetazidine dihydrochloride, 1-(2,3,4-trimethoxybenzyl) piperazine dihydrochloride

　　Structural formula:

　　Molecular formula: $C_{14}H_{22}N_2O_3 \cdot 2HCl$

　　Molecular weight: 339.3

[Description] This medicine is film coated

[Indications]

　　This drug can prevent angina pectoris. It can assist in the treatment of vertigo and tinnitus as well.

[Strength] 20mg

[Dosage and administration]

　　Take one tablet three times a day after meals

[Adverse reactions]

　　Generally, there is no obvious discomfort, and some individual might have intestinal reaction (such as nausea and allergic reactions).

[Contraindications]

　　This drug is not allowed to be used in allergic person and the women who are in lactating period.

[Precautions]

　　This drug can not directly treat angina, but has auxiliary effect on the treatment of angina.

[Pregnancy and lactation]

According to the data of animal experiments, there was no case of embryo malformation. But this does not mean there is no risk for human. Therefore, pregnant women are not recommended to use this drug.

[Use in Breastfeeding and Children]

No relevant experimental data can prove whether this drug and its metabolism will appear in the breast milk, lactating women should not use this drug.

[Interactions of drugs]

If you are receiving other treatment, you must use the medicine according to the doctor's order.

[Over dosage]

Always follow the doctor's instruction about the dosage of this drug. To avoid adverse reactions of the drug, it is forbidden to increase the drug dosage without doctor's permission.

[Pharmacology]

Protects energy metabolism in cells under the condition of oxygen deficiency to maintain a constant level of intracellular ATP.

In animals:

Trimetazidine:

- Keep the energy metabolism in the heart and neuro sensory organs at normal level.

- Maintain the constant concentration of intracellular and extracellular ions.

- Avoid the migration and infiltration of polynuclear neutrophils during the period of the myocardial ischemia.

In man:

Controlled studies in angina patients have shown that trimetazidine:

- Increase the blood flow of coronary artery, reduce the occurrence of ischemia.

- Reduce the rapid fluctuation of blood pressure, no effect on heart rate.

- Reduce the attack frequency of angina pectoris remarkably.

- Reduce the consumption of nitroglycerin.

[Pharmacokinetics]

the peak plasma concentration is about 35ng/ml.

- During repeated administration，the steady state is reached after 24 to 36 hours and remains very stable throughout treatment.

- The time needed to reach the plasma peak of this drug is less than 2 hours.

- The plasma peak concentration of this drug is 35ng/ml.

- This drug is primarily eliminated in the form of urine.

- The half-life is about 6 hours.

〔**Storage**〕 below 25℃

〔**Package**〕 15，30，60 tablets/box

〔**Shelf life**〕 24 months

Vocabulary（课文词汇）

insert 药品说明书

ingredient 成分

description 性状

indication 适应证

dosage 剂量

administration 用法

adverse reaction 不良反应

contraindication 禁忌证

precaution 注意事项

pregnancy 孕妇

lactation 哺乳期妇女

interaction of drugs 药物间作用

pharmacology 药理作用

film-coated 薄膜包衣

pharmacokinetics 药代动力学

approval 批准

Quiz（课后检测）

Answer the questions after reading the following insert.

Insert of Trimetazidine Dihydrochloride Tablets

〔**Dosage and administration**〕

Take one tablet three times a day after meals

[Adverse reactions]

Generally, there is no obvious discomfort, and some individual might have intestinal reaction (such as nausea and allergic reactions).

[Storage] below 25℃

[Package] Alu-Alu blister; 15,30,60 tablets/box

[Shelf life] 24 months

1. The Chinese meaning of the insert is _____.

2. Translate this English insertinto Chinese.

Discussion（问题讨论）

- How many expressions are there about the drug instruction in English?

- How many items in the imported drug instruction are there?

- What is the meaning of the description?

- What is the meaning of the dosage and administration?

Reading Material（延伸阅读）

Description of Ofloxacin

（氧氟沙星说明书）

Ofloxacin belongs to quinolones, which is a kind of broad-spectrum antibiotics. This drug can interfere with the function of DNA enzyme and inhibit the reproduction of bacteria or virus. It can inhibit many kinds of pathogenic bacteria. It is mainly used to treat the common acute and chronic infections caused by gram-negative bacteria, such as pneumonia, otitis media, enteritis, etc.

Cautions in application of Ofloxacin
（氧氟沙星应用注意事项）

It is not suitable for children under 18 years old. Patients with severe renal insufficiency，epilepsy and cerebral arteriosclerosis should use this drug with caution. Dosage should be adjusted in the elderly and those with renal insufficiency. Drink more water during medication and avoid overexposure to the sun.

Unit 4

Biopharmaceutics
第四单元　生物制药

> **Study Objective**（学习目标）
>
> 1. Grasping the pharmaceutical English terms.
> 2. Learning how to translate pharmaceutical English.
> 3. Getting familiar with the important knowledge of raw materials for medicine production.

Part 1　The Foundations of Biochemistry
第一部分　生物化学基础
Lesson 13　Amino Acids and Proteins
第十三课　氨基酸和蛋白质

Situational Entry（情境导入）

The organism continues to produce a variety of substances related to the regulation and metabolism of organisms, such as proteins, enzymes, nucleic acids, hormones, antibodies, cell and other factors. This makes the normal body can maintain healthy and have the ability to withstand and overcome the disease. Their regulatory roles help us maintain the normal function of the living body. According to this feature of these substances, we can extract them from the organisms as drug raw materials.

Proteins are the most abundant biological macromolecules，occurring in all cells and all parts of cells. Proteins also occur in great variety；thousands of different kinds，ranging in size from relatively small peptides to huge polymers with molecular weights in the millions，may be found in a single cell. Moreover，proteins exhibit an enormous diversity of biological function and are the most important final products of the information pathways discussed in this topic.

Information about proteins（蛋白质的相关知识）

What are proteins?（什么是蛋白质？）

Proteins are large biological molecules，or macromolecules，consisting of one or more long chains of amino acid residues linked together through peptide bonds. Each protein is made from the 20 standard amino acids and fold into a specific structure.

What do proteins do in the organism?（蛋白质在生物体中的作用有哪些？）

Proteins perform a vast array of functions within living organisms，including catalyzing metabolic reactions，replicating DNA，responding to stimuli，and transporting molecules from one location to another. Proteins differ from one another primarily in their sequence of amino acids，which is dictated by the nucleotide sequence of their genes，and which usually results in folding of the protein into a specific three-dimensional structure that determines its activity.

Molecular composition of proteins（蛋白质的分子组成）

Major elements：C($50\%\sim55\%$)，H($\sim7\%$)，O($19\%\sim20\%$)，N($13\%\sim19\%$)，S($\sim4\%$). The average nitrogen content in proteins is about 16%，and proteins are the major source of N in biological systems. The protein quantity can be estimated.

Trace elements：P，Fe，Cu，Zn，I.

Amino acids（AAs）——basic building blocks of proteins（氨基酸——蛋白质的基本组成单位）

Ionization of amino acids（氨基酸的电离）：

An amino group，a carboxyl group，an H atom and an R group are connected to a C atom (Fig. 13-1). The R groups are different in 20 AAs. There are about 300 types of AAs in nature, but only 20 types are used for protein synthesis in biological systems. These 20 AAs belong to L-α-amino acids except glycine (Fig. 13-2).

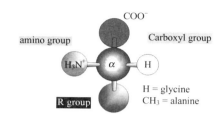

Fig. 13-1   Composition of amino acids

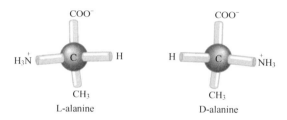

Fig. 13-2   L-α-amino acids and D-α-amino acids

Molecular weight（分子量）

The mass of proteins is expressed in units of Daltons. Most natural proteins contain between 50 and 2000 amino acids. The average molecular weight of most amino acids is about 110. A protein with a molecular weight of 50,000 has a mass of 50,000 Daltons, or 50kDa (kilo-Daltons).

Isoelectric point, pI（等电点）

The pH at which an amino acid exists as zwitterions with no net charge is called isoelectric point (given the symbol pI) (Fig. 13-3). When pH$>$pI, protein moves toward anode. When pH$<$pI, protein moves toward cathode. When pH$=$pI, no migrate.

Peptide and peptide bond（肽和肽键）

Peptide is the compound that the amino acids joined through the peptide bonds to yield. Peptide bond is a covalent bond formed by removal of the elements of water (dehydration) from the carboxyl group of one amino acid and the α-amino group of another (Fig. 13-4).

$$
\underset{\substack{\text{COOH}\\|\\H_3N^+-C-H\\|\\R}}{}
\quad
\overset{-H^+}{\underset{+H^+}{\overset{pK_1'}{\rightleftharpoons}}}
\quad
\underset{\substack{\text{COO}^-\\|\\H_3N^+-C-H\\|\\R}}{}
\quad
\overset{-H^+}{\underset{+H^+}{\overset{pK_2'}{\rightleftharpoons}}}
\quad
\underset{\substack{\text{COO}^-\\|\\H_2N-C-H\\|\\R}}{}
$$

pH	1	7	10
net charge	+1	0	−1
	cation	zwitterion	anion
		pI	

Fig. 13-3   The isoelectric point of proteins

$$
\underset{\substack{H\;\;\;O\\|\;\;\;\|\\H_2N-C-C-OH}}{\underset{\substack{|\\R^1}}{}}
\;\;\;
\underset{\substack{H\\|\\H-N-C-COOH}}{\underset{\substack{|\\R^2}}{}}
\;\;\longrightarrow\;\;
\underset{\substack{H\;\;\;O\;\;\;\;\;H\\|\;\;\;\|\;\;\;\;\;|\\H_2N-C-C-HN-C-COOH}}{\underset{\substack{|\;\;\;\;\;\;\;\;\;\;\;|\\R^1\;\;\;\;\;\;\;\;R^2}}{}}
$$

H_2O

peptide bond

Fig. 13-4   The peptide bond of the proteins

Dipeptide：2 amino acid residues，oligopeptide：2～10 amino acid residues，polypeptide：>10 amino acid residues，protein：molecular weight>10kDa.

The molecular structure of proteins（蛋白质的分子结构）（Fig. 13-5）

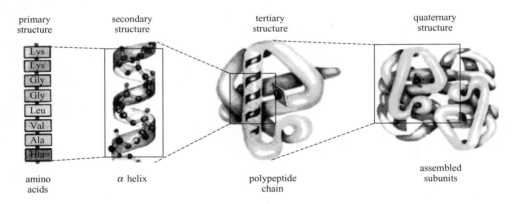

Fig. 13-5   The structure of the proteins

The primary structure（一级结构）

The most important element of the primary structure is the sequence of amino acid residues. A linear chain of amino acid residues is called a polypeptide. A protein contains at least one long polypeptide. A polypeptide chain consisted of a regularly repeating part is called the main chain，and a variable part comprises the distinctive side chains. By convention，the amine end（N terminal）of an amino acid is always on the left，while the acid end（C terminal）is on the right.

Secondary structure（二级结构）

The term secondary structure refers to the local conformation of some part of a polypeptide. The discussion of secondary structure most usefully focuses on common regular folding patterns of the polypeptide backbone. Main patterns of the secondary structure of a protein are：α-helix （α-螺旋），β-pleated sheet （β-折叠），β-turn （β-转角），and random coil （无规卷曲）. Hydrogen bonds （氢键） are responsible for stabilizing the secondary structure.

Tertiary structure（三级结构）

The term tertiary structure refers to the overall three-dimensional arrangement of all atoms in a protein.

Quaternary structure（四级结构）

Quaternary structure is defined as the spatial arrangement of multiple subunits of a protein.

Proteins need to have two or more polypeptide chains to function properly. Each individual peptide is called subunit. These subunits are associated with H-bonds，ionic interactions，and hydrophobic interactions. Polypeptide chains can be in dimer，trimer，etc.

Applications（应用实例）

Human plasma contains many proteins with different structures and functions，such as albumin，globulin，and fibrinogen，which play important role in the formation of colloid osmotic pressure，water distribution of the regulating inside and outside the vessel，participating in the immune response. With the development of blood transfusion therapy，people recognized the input of the plasma component has a therapeutic effect on many diseases. The attempting on the separating and purification the target protein from plasma has made a great progress，such as gamma globulin （γ- globulin），serum albumin，plasma coagulation factor.

Vocabulary（课文词汇）

protein 蛋白质
trace element 微量元素
amino acid residue 氨基酸残基
macromolecule 大分子

peptide bond 肽键

atom 原子

molecular weight 分子量

dalton 道尔顿

isoelectric point 等电点

zwitterion 两性离子

charge 电荷

dipeptide 二肽

oligopeptide 寡肽

polypeptide 多肽

primary structure 一级结构

secondary structure 二级结构

tertiary structure 三级结构

quaternary structure 四级结构

dimer 二聚体

trimer 三聚体

Summary（重点小结）

1. Proteins are large biological molecules，or macromolecules，consisting of one or more long chains of amino acid residues linked together through peptide bonds.

2. The average nitrogen content in proteins is about 16％，and proteins are the major source of N in biological systems.

3. A linear chain of amino acid residues is called a polypeptide. A protein contains at least one long polypeptide.

4. Main patterns of the secondary structure of a protein：α-helix（α-螺旋），β-pleated sheet（β-折叠），β-turn（β-转角），random coil（无规卷曲）.

5. Hydrogen bonds（氢键）are responsible for stabilizing the secondary structure.

6. Proteins need to have two or more polypeptide chains to function properly.

Quiz（课后检测）

Ⅰ. **Fill in the blanks according to the information about proteins.**

1. The pH at which an amino acid exists as zwitterions with no net charge is called _____ .

2. Many amino acids joined by peptide bonds are called a _____ .

3. A polypeptide chain consisted of a regularly repeating part is called the _____ , and a variable part comprises the distinctive _____ .

4. The mass of proteins is expressed in units of _____ .

Ⅱ. **Give the proper explanation on the glycine according to the following picture.**

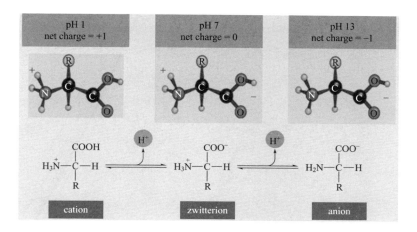

Discussion（问题讨论）

- What is responsible for stabilizing the primary structure of proteins?
- What is responsible for stabilizing the secondary structure of proteins?
- How many main patterns of the secondary structure of the protein are there in the world?
- Why do the proteins can be used to produce drugs?
- Lists protein-related diseases that you know.

Reading Material（延伸阅读）

Peptides are chains of amino acids
（肽是氨基酸组成的长链）

Two amino acid molecules can be covalently joined through a substituted amide linkage，termed a peptide bond，to yield a dipeptide. Such a linkage is formed by removal of the elements of water（dehydration）from the carboxyl group of one amino acid and the amino group of another. Peptide bond formation is an example of a condensation reaction，a common class of reactions in living cells. Under standard biochemical conditions，the equilibrium for the reaction shown in favors the amino acids over the dipeptide. To make the reaction thermodynamically more favorable, the carboxyl group must be chemically modified or activated so that the hydroxyl group can be more readily eliminated. Three amino acids can be joined by two peptide bonds to form a tripeptide; similarly, amino acids can be linked to form tetrapeptides, pentapeptides, and so forth. When a few amino acids are joined in this fashion, the structure is called an oligopeptide. When many amino acids are joined, the product is called a polypeptide. Proteins may have thousands of amino acid residues. Although the terms "protein" and "polypeptide" are sometimes used interchangeably, molecules referred to as polypeptides generally have molecular weights below 10,000, and those called proteins have higher molecular weights.

Lesson 14 Nucleic Acids
第十四课 核酸

Situational Entry（情境导入）

Nucleic acids were named for their initial discovery within the nucleus，and for the presence of phosphate groups (related to phosphoric acid). Although first discovered within the nucleus of eukaryotic cells，nucleic acids are now known to be found in all life forms as well as some nonliving entities，including bacteria，archaea，mitochondria，chloroplasts，viruses and viroids. All living cells contain both DNA and RNA（except some cells such as mature red blood cells），while viruses contain either DNA or RNA，but usually not both. There are a lot of nucleic acid drugs（Fig. 14-1）.

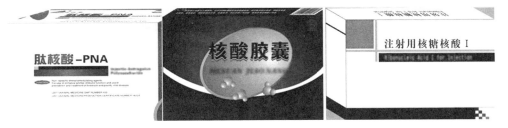

Fig. 14-1　The drugs produced by nucleic acids as raw materials

Information about nucleic acids（核酸的相关知识）

What is nucleic acid? （什么是核酸?）

Nucleic acids are polymeric macromolecules，or large biological molecules，essential for all known forms of life. Nucleic acids，including DNA（deoxyribo-nucleic acid）and RNA（ribonucleic acid），are made from monomers known as nucleotides.

Classification of nucleic acid （核酸的分类）

Ribonucleic acid （RNA）

RNA is made by copying the base sequence of a section of double-stranded DNA，gene，into a piece of single-stranded nucleic acid. The main function is to realize the expression of genetic information on the protein. It is a bridge in the process of genetic information to phenotypic transformation.

Deoxyribonucleic acid（DNA）

The DNA molecule consists of two strands that wind around one another to form a shape known as a double helix. It exists in the nucleus，the function of DNA is to store genetic information.

Nucleotide——basic unit of nucleic acid（核苷酸——核酸的基本组成单位）

A nucleotide consists of three parts（a nitrogenous base，a pentose，a phosphate group）. If the sugar is deoxyribose，the polymer is DNA. If the sugar is ribose，the polymer is RNA（Fig. 14-2）. A nucleic acid chain，having a phosphate group at $5'$ end and α-OH group at $3'$ end，can only be extended from the $3'$ end，forming a $5'$-$3'$ phosphodiester bond.

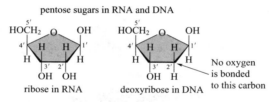

Fig. 14-2   The pentose of the nucleic acid

Components of nucleic acids（核酸的组成成分）

The bases in the nucleotides are nitrogen-containing heterocyclic compounds，which are composed of pyrimidine and purine. Adenine，guanine and cytosine，thymine mainly exist in DNA. Adenine，guanine and cytosine，and uracil are mainly present in RNA. There are two kinds of pentose DNA in nucleic acid：D-2-deoxyribose（D-2-deoxyribose）in DNA and D-ribose（D-ribose）in RNA（Fig. 14-3）.

Together with proteins，nucleic acids are the most important biological macromolecules. They are found abundant in all living things，where they function in encoding，transmitting and expressing genetic information. In other words，information is conveyed through the nucleic acid sequence，or the order of nucleotides within a DNA or RNA molecule. Strings of nucleotides strung together in a specific sequence are the mechanism for storing and transmitting hereditary，or genetic information via protein synthesis.

Structure of nucleic acid（核酸的结构）

The primary structure of nucleic acid（核酸的一级结构）

In the primary structure of DNA，A，C，G，and T are linked by $3'$-$5'$ ester

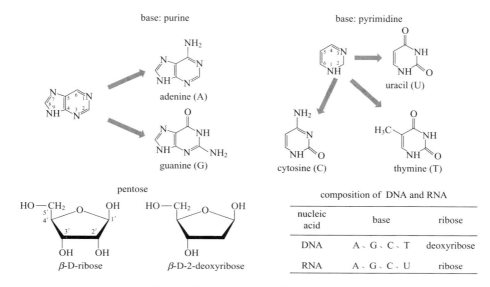

Fig. 14-3   The composition of the nucleic acid

bonds between deoxyribose and phosphate. The primary structure of RNA is a single strand of nucleotides. It consists of the bases A，C，G，and U linked by 3′-5′ ester bonds between ribose and phosphate（Fig. 14-4）.

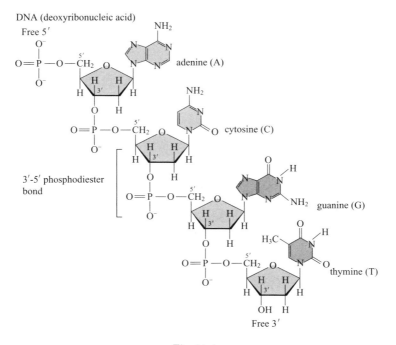

Fig. 14-4

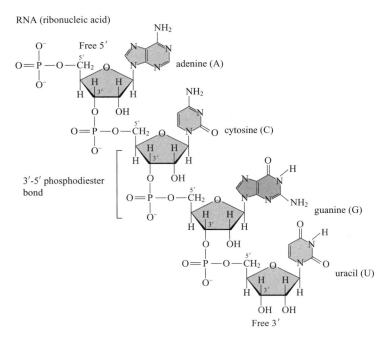

RNA (ribonucleic acid)

Fig. 14-4   The structure of the nucleic acid

The secondary structure of nucleic acid（核酸的二级结构）

The DNA structure is a double helix like a spiral staircase that consists of two strands of nucleotides. Hydrogen bonds between the bases A-T and G-C is the main force of the secondary structure.

Classification of RNA （RNA 的分类）

mRNA （messenger RNA）：mRNA is the template for protein synthesis，to translate each genetic codon on mRNA into each AA in proteins. Each genetic codon is a set of three continuous nucleotides on mRNA.

tRNA （transfer RNA）：tRNA serves as an amino acid carrier to transport AA for protein synthesis.

rRNA （ribosomal RNA）：a component of ribosome for protein synthesis.

hnRNA （heterogeneous nuclear RNA）：precursor of mRNA.

snRNA （small nuclei RNA）：small RNAs for processing and transporting hnRNA.

Human genome project （人类基因组计划）

Completed in 2003，the human genome project （HGP） was a 13-year project coordinated by the U. S. Department of Energy and the National Institutes of Health. During the early years of the HGP, the Welcome Trust (U. K.) became a major partner. Additional contributions came from Japan, France, Germany, China, and other countries.

Mutation (突变)

The gene is very stable. It can reproduce itself accurately when the cell divides. But this stability is relative. Under certain conditions, the gene can suddenly change from the original form to another new one. That is, a new gene suddenly appears on one site, replacing the original gene. Gene mutation refers to the change of the gene in the cell (usually the deoxyribonucleic acid exists in the nucleus). It includes a point mutation caused by a single base change, or deletion, duplication and insertion of multiple bases. The reason is that the genetic duplication of cells is wrong, or is influenced by chemicals, radiation or viruses. Mutations usually lead to abnormal or death of cells, and even lead to cancer in higher organisms. The normal DNA sequence produces a mRNA that provides instructions for the correct series of amino acids in a protein [Fig. 14-5(a)]. The altered sequence of genes is unable to complete the translation process, such as insertions or deletions of a nucleotide (mutation) [Fig. 14-5(b)].

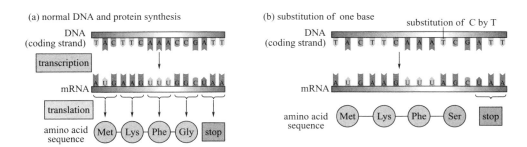

Fig. 14-5   The genetic mutations of the nucleic acid

Vocabulary (课文词汇)

nucleic acid 核酸

monomer 单体

deoxyribose 脱氧核糖

ribose 核糖

polymeric 聚合的

nucleotide 核苷酸

nitrogenous base 含氮碱基

genome 基因组

mitochondria 线粒体

chloroplast 叶绿体

pentose 戊糖

purine 嘌呤

phosphodiester bonds 磷酸二酯键

codon 密码

Summary（重点小结）

1. Nucleic acids are polymeric macromolecules，or large biological molecules，including DNA（deoxyribonucleic acid）and RNA（ribonucleic acid），are made from monomers known as nucleotides.

2. A nucleotide consists of three parts（a nitrogenous base，a pentose，a phosphate group）.

3. In the primary structure of DNA，A，C，G，and T are linked by $3'$-$5'$ ester bonds between deoxyribose and phosphate.

4. The primary structure of RNA is a single strand of nucleotides. It consists of the bases A，C，G，and U linked by $3'$-$5'$ ester bonds between ribose and phosphate.

5. The human genome project（HGP）was a 13-year project coordinated by the U. S. department of Energy and the National Institutes of Health.

6. RNA includes mRNA，tRNA and hnRNA.

Quiz（课后检测）

Ⅰ. Fill in the blanks according to the information about nucleic acids.

1. If the sugar is deoxyribose，the polymer is _____ . If the sugar is ribose，the polymer is _____ .

2. _____ serves as an amino acid carrier to transport AA for protein synthesis.

3. _____ bonds between the bases A–T and G–C is the main force of the secondary structure.

4. The DNA structure is a double _____ that consists of two strands of nucleotides.

Ⅱ. **Answer the questions according to the diagram.**

A. Give the name and abbreviation for the following and list its nitrogen base and sugar.

B. Write the complementary base sequence for the matching strand in the following DNA section：

Discussion（问题讨论）

- Why do the nucleic acids can be used to produce the drugs?
- What is the application of nucleic acid?
- What is the difference between DNA and RNA in composition?
- What is the difference between DNA and RNA in structure?
- What type of bond is found between the bases in a DNA molecule?

Reading Material（延伸阅读）

DNA map
（基因图谱）

DNA is the whole "map" of the human body. It is something that all humans have，and it tells the body what to do. We look like our parents because we get some of their DNA to make our own. People have been trying to understand the human body for a long time. In 1860，Mr. Mendel discovered why we look the same as other people in our family. It is because of small things called "genes" （基因）in our body. In 1953，two scientists，Watson and Crick，found out that those small parts are really messages. They're written in the DNA with a special language. In 1961，other two scientists found the first "word" that they could understand in that language. It shows how DNA tells the cell （细胞）to build its parts. By understanding what just one "word" means，we can help to save people from several illnesses. So the more we understand，the more doctors will be able to do.

Most people hope that this will help to make better medicine and help sick people. However，other people worry that when we learn more "words" and find out more information，we will use it in the wrong way.

Lesson 15 Polysaccharides
第十五课 多糖

🎙 Situational Entry（情境导入）

Saccharide is another name for carbohydrate. Simple saccharides are the monosaccharides，commonly called sugars. Saccharides are the most abundant biomolecules on Earth. Each year，photosynthesis converts more than 100 billion metric tons of CO_2 and H_2O into cellulose and other plant products. Certain carbohydrates（sugar and starch）are a dietary staple in most parts of the world，and the oxidation of carbohydrates is the central energy-yielding pathway in most nonphotosynthetic cells. The biggest feature of the most saccharide-based drugs（Fig. 15-1）has a direct effect on the cell surface. They do not enter the interior of the cell with the small injury on the body. Most saccharide-based drugs play a vital role in anti-tumor.

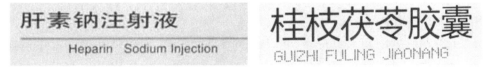

Fig. 15-1   The drugs produced by saccharides as raw materials

Information about polysaccharides（多糖的相关知识）

What are the saccharides?（什么是糖类？）

Saccharides are simply defined as polyhydroxy aldehydes or ketones and their derivatives. Many have the empirical formula（CH_2O）$_n$，which originally suggested they were "hydrates" of carbon. There are three major size classes of carbohydrates：monosaccharides，oligosaccharides，and polysaccharides（the word "saccharide" is derived from the Greek sakcharon，meaning "sugar"）.

Polysaccharides（多糖）

They are polymers of monosaccharide units. The monomeric units of a polysaccharide are usually all the same (called homopolysaccharides), though there are exceptions (called heteropolysaccharides). Examples include chondroitin sulfates, keratan sulfates, dermatan sulfates, hyaluronic acid, heparin.

Some polysaccharides, such as cellulose, are linear chains; others, such as glycogen, are branched. Animals use glycogen. Plants use starch, which is composed of amylose and amylopectin. In both plants and animals, the polysaccharides used for energy storage are readily broken down into monomeric units that can be rapidly metabolized to produce ATP. In addition to polysaccharides used for energy storage, plants use different polysaccharides, such as cellulose, for structural purposes in their cell walls.

Application（应用实例）

In recent years, with the development of molecular pharmacology, we found that many clinical drugs produce utility by acting on the sugar molecule, such as some of the antibiotics erythromycin, vancomycin etc. There have been a large number of biopharmaceutical companies devoting to the development of carbohydrate drugs, including GlycoDesign (Toronto, ON, Canada)、Biomira (Edmonton, AB, Canada)、GlycoTech (Rockville, MD, USA)、Neose Technologies (Horsham, PA, USA).

Heparin is one of the most common anti-clotting drugs. It is a kind of mucopolysaccharide that consists of sulfuric acid D-glucosamine, D-glucuronide, and low molecular weight heparin (LMWH) (Fig. 15-2).

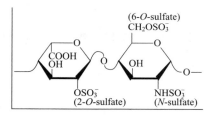

Fig. 15-2　The structure of the heparin

Vocabulary（课文词汇）

saccharide 糖类

polysaccharides 多糖

homopolysaccharides 均一多糖

heteropolysaccharides 非均一多糖

chondroitin sulfate 硫酸软骨素

keratan sulfate 硫酸角质素

dermatan sulfate 硫酸皮肤素

hyaluronic acid 透明质酸

heparin 肝素

cellulose 纤维素

glycogen 糖原

anti-clotting 抗凝血

Summary（重点小结）

1. Saccharides are simply defined as polyhydroxy aldehydes or ketones and their derivatives.

2. The monomeric units of a polysaccharide are usually all the same（called homopolysaccharides）.

3. Examples of heteropolysaccharides include chondroitin sulfates，keratan sulfates，dermatan sulfates，hyaluronic acid，heparin.

Quiz（课后检测）

Fill in the blanks according to the information about saccharides.

1. Polysaccharides used for energy _____ . Animals use _____ . Plants use _____ .

2. The most abundant monosaccharide in nature is the six-carbon sugar _____ .

Discussion（问题讨论）

• Why do the saccharides can be used to produce drugs?

• What is the difference between homopolysaccharides and heteropolysaccharides?

• What is the contribution of the polysaccharides to society?

Reading Material（延伸阅读）

Cellulose transform into starch
（纤维素转化为淀粉）

A team of Virginia Tech researchers has succeeded in transforming cellulose（纤维素）into starch（淀粉），a process that has the potential to provide a previously untapped nutrient source from plants that were not traditionally thought of as food crops. Y. H. Percival Zhang，an associate professor of biological systems engineering in the College of Agriculture and Life Sciences and the College of Engineering，led a team of researchers in the project that could help feed a growing global population that is estimated to increase to 9 billion by 2050. Starch is one of the most important components of the human diet and provides $20\% \sim 40\%$ of our daily caloric intake.

The research was published in the early edition of the Proceedings of the National Academy of Sciences. Cellulose is the supporting material in plant cell walls and is the most common carbohydrate on Earth. This new development opens the door to the potential that food could be created from any plant，reducing the need for crops to be grown on valuable land that requires fertilizers，pesticides，and large amount of water. The type of starch that Zhang's team produced is amylose，a linear resistant starch that is not broken down in the digestion process and acts as a good source of dietary fiber. It has been proven to decrease the risk of obesity and diabetes.

This discovery holds promise on many fronts beyond food systems. "Besides serving as a food source，the starch can be used in the manufacture of edible，clear films for biodegradable food packaging," Zhang said. "It can even serve as a high-density hydrogen storage carrier that could solve problems related to hydrogen storage and distribution."

Zhang used a novel process involving cascading enzymes to transform cellulose into amylose starch. "Cellulose and starch have the same chemical formula," Zhang said. "The difference is in their chemical linkages. Our idea is to use an enzyme cascade to break up the bonds in cellulose，enabling their reconfiguration as starch."

The new approach takes cellulose from non-food plant material，such as corn stover, converts about 30% to amylose, and hydrolyzes the remainder to glucose suitable for ethanol production. Corn stover consists of the stem, leaves, and husk of the corn plant remaining after ears of corn are harvested. Even better, the process works with cellulose from any plant.

This bioprocess called "simultaneous enzymatic biotransformation and microbial fermentation（发酵）" is easy to scale up for commercial production. It is environmental friendly because it does not require expensive equipment, heat, or chemical reagents, and does not generate any waste. The key enzymes immobilized on the magnetic nanoparticles can easily be recycled using a magnetic force.

Lesson 16　Lipids
第十六课　脂类

Situational Entry（情境导入）

　　Lipids are fat and fat-like organic substance that widely exists in the living body，with the high ratio of the hydrocarbon molecules. They can be dissolved in organic solvents，such as ether（乙醚），chloroform（氯仿），benzene（苯），etc.，and insoluble in water. Such properties of lipid compounds are called fat-soluble. We can extract the lipids from the organism with an organic solvent according to the feature of lipids. Lipids are used to produce supplement such as lecithin，CoQ10，DHA capsule，etc.

Information about lipids（脂类的相关知识）

What are lipids?（什么是脂类？）

　　Lipids are compounds insoluble in water and can be extracted by nonpolar organic solvents such as ethyl ether，chloroform and benzene. It is composed of fatty acids，alcohols，esters and their derivatives. There are three types of molecules that fall under the category of "lipids"，including triglycerides（甘油三酯），phospholipids（磷脂）and sterols（固醇）(Fig. 16-1).

Triglyceride（甘油三酯）

　　Triglycerides consist of three molecules of fatty acids and one molecule of glycerol. The molecule of glycerol is relatively simple，but the type and length of fatty acids are complicated. Triglyceride is the lipid with the highest content in human body，and most tissues can be supplied with energy by triglyceride decomposition products. The ideal triglyceride level should be lower than 1.70mmol/L. If it exceeds 1.70mmol/L，people need to change lifestyle，control diet and increase exercise. If it is higher than 2.26mmol/L，it means the triglyceride level is too high and medicine is needed to prevent pathological changes.

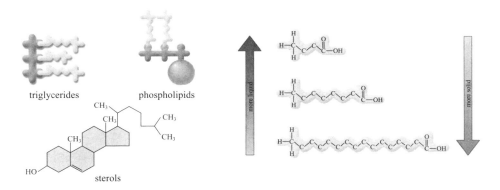

triglycerides   phospholipids

sterols

Fig. 16-1   The types of lipids

Fatty acids（脂肪酸）

What is fatty acids?（什么是脂肪酸？）

Fatty acids are carboxylic acids with long hydrocarbon chains. Most fatty acids contain even carbon atoms because they are usually biosynthesized from two carbon units. There are about 40 different kinds of fatty acids in nature. The physical properties of many lipids depend on the saturation of fatty acids and the length of carbon chains, of which only even carbon atoms can be absorbed and utilized by the human body.

The classification of fatty acids（脂肪酸的分类）

Fatty acids are classified into three types according to the length of carbon chain, short chain fatty acids（containing 2～4 carbon atoms）, medium chain fatty acids（containing 6～12 carbon atoms）and long chain fatty acids（containing more than 14 carbon atoms）.

Fatty acids are straight chain hydrocarbons possessing a carboxyl（—COOH）group at one end, which may or may not contain carbon-carbon double bonds. Fatty acids can be classified into three groups according to the saturation of hydrocarbon chains. Saturated fatty acids are fatty acids without carbon-carbon double bonds. The unsaturated fatty acids are further divided into monounsaturated fatty acids and polyunsaturated fatty acids according to the degree of unsaturation. Monounsaturated fatty acids are fatty acids with a carbon-carbon double bond. Polyunsaturated fatty acids are fatty acids with two or more carbon-carbon double bonds（Fig. 16-2）and 18 to 22 carbon atoms in length, which are classified into omega-3 and omega-6 fatty acids. The omega-3 fatty acids are also called ω-3 fatty acids or n-3 fatty acids. The omega-6 fatty acids are also called ω-6 fatty acids or n-6 fatty acids.

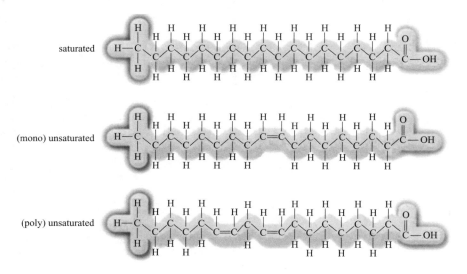

Fig. 16-2   The structure of fatty acids

Saturated fats are typically solids and are derived from animals, while unsaturated fats are liquids and usually extracted from plants. Unsaturated fats assume a particular geometry that prevents the molecules from packing as efficiently as they do in saturated molecules. Thus the boiling points of unsaturated fats are lower. If the number of carbon atoms is an even number, the fatty acids are usually unbranched.

Fatty acids can also be classified into essential fatty acids and non-essential fatty acids according to the needs of the human body. Nonessential fatty acids are fatty acids that can be synthesized by the body and do not depend on food supply. They include saturated fatty acids and some monounsaturated fatty acids. Essential fatty acids, or EFAs, are fatty acids that humans and other animals must ingest because the body requires them for good health but cannot synthesize them. All of them are unsaturated fatty acids, belonging to omega 3 and omega 6 polyunsaturated fatty acids, such as alpha-linolenic acid（亚麻酸）（an omega-3 fatty acid) and linoleic acid（亚油酸）（an omega-6 fatty acid).

Some other fatty acids are sometimes classified as "conditionally essential", meaning that they can become essential under some developmental or disease conditions. Examples include docosahexaenoic acid（二十二碳六烯酸）（an omega-3 fatty acid) and gamma-linolenic acid（次亚麻酸）（an omega-6 fatty acid）.

Other products and utility（其他产品及用途）

The ketone body（acetone bodies）is a special intermediate product produced by the normal catabolism of fatty acids in the liver，including acetoacetic acid （～30％），beta hydroxybutyric acid（～70％）and a very small amount of acetone. Normal human blood has a small amount of ketone body，this is normal due to the body's use of fat oxidation as an energy supply. However，under certain physiological conditions（hunger，fasting）or pathological conditions（such as diabetes），the source of sugar or oxidative energy supply is obstructed and lipid mobilization is enhanced，fatty acid becomes the main energy supply in the body. If the amount of ketone body in the liver is more than the ability of the liver tissue to use，resulting in ketonemia（acetonemia）and ketonuria（acetonuria）. Acetoacetic acid and beta hydroxybutyric acid are both acidic substances，so ketone bodies accumulate in bulk and cause acidosis.

Applications（应用实例）

Polyunsaturated fatty acids（PUFAs）belong to the essential fatty acids. Many scientists found that the rate of the coronary heart of Eskimo people in Greenland is significantly lower than other areas. This is because their food is full of n-3 PUFAs that has a protective effect on the cardiovascular system. Eicosapentaenoic acid （EPA）and docosahexaenoic acid（DHA）from deep-sea fish and fish oil are not only a food ingredient but also a drug ingredient. They appeared in many high purity n-3 PUFAs drugs.

Vocabulary（课文词汇）

lipid 脂类
chloroform 氯仿、三氯甲烷
fatty acid 脂肪酸
cholesterol 胆固醇
steroid 类固醇
phospholipid 磷脂
polyunsaturated 多不饱和的

Summary（重点小结）

1. Lipids are molecules that contain hydrocarbons and make up the building blocks of the structure and function of living cells.

2. Fatty acids are straight chain hydrocarbons possessing a carboxyl（—COOH）group at one end，which may or may not contain carbon-carbon double bonds.

3. Fatty acids can also be classified into essential fatty acids and non-essential fatty acids according to the needs of the human body.

4. Under certain physiological conditions（hunger，fasting）or pathological conditions（such as diabetes），the source of sugar or oxidative energy supply is obstructed and lipid mobilization is enhanced，fatty acid becomes the main energy supply in the body.

Quiz（课后检测）

Fill in the blanks according to the information about lipids.

1. There are three types of molecules that fall under the category of "lipids"，including _____，_____，_____ .

2. _____ are fatty acids without carbon-carbon double bonds.

3. _____ fatty acids，or EFAs，are fatty acids that humans and other animals must ingest because the body requires them for good health but cannot synthesize them.

Discussion（问题讨论）

- Why can the lipids be used to produce drugs?
- What is the application of lipids?
- What are the essential fatty acids?

Reading Material（延伸阅读）

Omega-3 fatty acids may give a boost to behavior，mood，and personality
（ω-3 脂肪酸有助于改善人的行为、情绪和个性）

Heart-healthy omega-3 fatty acids，like those found in fish，may give a boost to behavior, mood and personality, new research suggests. University of Pittsburgh researchers found that volunteers with lower levels of omega-3 polyunsaturated fatty acids in blood were more likely than others to be impulsive, to have a more negative outlook, and to report mild or moderate symptoms of depression. Study participants with higher levels of omega-3 fatty acids in blood were found to be more agreeable, however. The findings were presented at the American Psychosomatic Society meeting, in Denver. "A number of previous studies have linked lower levels of omega-3 to clinically significant conditions such as major depressive disorder, bipolar disorder, schizophrenia, substance abuse and attention-deficit disorder." Sarah Conklin, a postdoctoral scholar with the psychiatry department's Cardiovascular Behavioral Medicine Program, said in prepared statement. "However, few studies have shown that these relationships also occur in healthy adults. This study opens the door for future research looking at what effect increasing omega-3 intake, whether by eating omega-3 rich foods like salmon, or taking fish-oil supplements, has on people's mood," Conklin said.

Lesson 17   Vitamins
第十七课   维生素

Situational Entry（情境导入）

Vitamins are necessary to maintain good health. The body will have a sudden illness when we are lack of them. Vitamin deficiency can cause disease，so vitamins play a very important role in the body (Fig. 17-1).

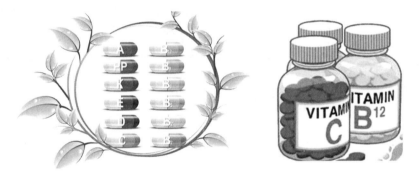

Fig. 17-1   The drugs produced by vitamins as raw materials

Information about vitamins（维生素的相关知识）

What are vitamins?（什么是维生素？）

Vitamins are a kind of trace organic substance that human and animals must obtain from food to maintain normal physiological functions and play an important role in growth，metabolism and development. Vitamins neither participate in the forming of human cells nor provide energy for the body.

The classification of vitamins（维生素的分类）

Based on the different solubility，the vitamins are divided into two groups，the fat-soluble vitamins and water-soluble vitamins. There are four fat-soluble vitamins，including A，D，E，and K. There are nine water-soluble vitamins which consist of the B vitamin complex and vitamin C.

Fat soluble-vitamins (脂溶性维生素)

Vitamin A is a fat-soluble vitamin. It can be found in many fruits, vegetables, eggs, whole milk, butter, fortified margarine, meat, and oily saltwater fish (Fig. 17-2). Vitamin A is important for normal vision, the immune system, and reproduction. Vitamin A also helps the heart, lungs, kidneys, and other organs work properly. Deficiency of vitamin A is the most common cause of non-accidental blindness.

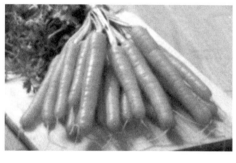

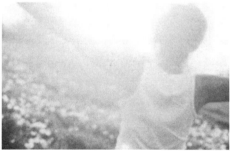

Fig. 17-2　The source of vitamin A and vitamin D

There are two different types of vitamin A. The first type, preformed vitamin A, is found in animal products. The second type, provitamin A, is found in plant-based products. The most common type of provitamin A in foods and dietary supplements is beta-carotene. In contrast to preformed vitamin A, beta-carotene is not toxic even at high levels of intake. The body can form vitamin A from beta-carotene as needed, and there is no need to monitor intake levels. Therefore, it is preferable to choose a multivitamin supplement that has all or the vast majority of its vitamin A in the form of beta-carotene. Many multivitamin manufacturers have already reduced the amount of preformed vitamin A in their products.

Vitamin D is an essential vitamin required by the body for the absorption of calcium, bone development, immune functioning, and alleviation of inflammation. Vitamin D has been called the new "wonder vitamin". Doctors are learning more and more about its role in good health and the prevention of diseases (Fig. 17-2). Unfortunately, most teens don't get enough. Vitamin D deficiency can lead to rickets, a weakened immune system, increased cancer risk, poor hair growth, and osteomalacia. Excess vitamin D can cause the body to absorb too much calcium, leading to increased risk of heart disease and kidney stones.

Water-soluble vitamins (水溶性维生素)

The B-group vitamins do not provide the body with fuel for energy, even though supplement advertisements often claim they do. It is true though that without B-group vitamins the body lacks energy. The body uses energy-yielding nutrients such as carbohydrates, fat and protein for fuel. The B-group vitamins help the body to use that fuel. Other B-group vitamins play necessary roles such as helping cells to multiply by making new DNA. Even though the B-group vitamins are found in many foods, they are water-soluble and delicate. They are easily destroyed, particularly by alcohol and cooking. The body has a limited capacity to store most of the B-group vitamins (except B_{12} and folate, which are stored in the liver). A person who has a poor diet for a few months may end up with B-group vitamins deficiency. For this reason, it is important that adequate amounts of these vitamins should be eaten regularly as part of a well-balanced, nutritious diet. There are eight types of vitamin B: thiamin (vitamin B_1), riboflavin, niacin, pantothenic acid, vitamin B_6 (pyridoxine), biotin (vitamin B_7), folate (called folic acid when included in supplements), vitamin B_{12} (cyanocobalamin).

Deficiencies (缺乏症)

Humans must consume vitamins periodically but with differing schedules, to avoid deficiency. The human body's storages for different vitamins vary widely. Vitamins A, D, and B_{12} are stored in significant amounts in the human body, mainly in the liver. An adult's diet may be deficient in vitamins A and D for many months and B_{12} in some cases for years, before developing a deficiency condition. However, vitamin B_3 (niacin and niacinamide) is not stored in significant amount, so the storage may last only a couple of weeks. The first symptoms of scurvy in experimental studies of complete vitamin C deprivation in humans have varied widely, from a month to more than six months, depending on previous dietary history that determined body storages.

Deficiencies of vitamins are classified as either primary or secondary. A primary deficiency occurs when an organism does not get enough vitamins in its food. A secondary deficiency may be due to an underlying disorder that prevents or limits the absorption or use of the vitamin, due to a "lifestyle factor", such as smoking, excessive alcohol consumption, or the use of medications that interfere with the absorption or use of the vitamin. People who eat a varied diet are unlikely to develop a severe primary vitamin deficiency. In contrast, restrictive diets have the potential to cause prolonged vitamin deficits, which may result in often painful and potentially deadly diseases. Well-known human vitamin deficiencies involve thiamine (beriberi), niacin (pellagra), vitamin C (scurvy), and vitamin D (rickets). In much of the developed world, such deficiencies are rare; this is due to an adequate supply of food and the addition of vitamins and minerals to common foods, often called fortification. In addition to these classical vitamin deficiency diseases, some evidence has also suggested links between vitamin deficiency and a number of different disorders.

Side-effects（副作用）

Some vitamins have documented side-effects that tend to be more severe with a larger dosage. The likelihood of consuming too much of any vitamin from food is minimal, but overdosing (vitamin poisoning) from vitamin supplementation does occur. At high enough dosages, some vitamins cause side-effects such as nausea, diarrhea, and vomiting. When side-effects happen, recovery is often accomplished by reducing the dosage. The doses of vitamins differ because individual tolerances can vary widely and appear to be related to age and state of health of individuals.

Applications（应用实例）

Vitamin drugs are mainly used to prevent and cure a variety of vitamin deficiency or to treat some diseases as an auxiliary. Large doses of vitamin also can be dangerous and，in some cases，life threatening.

Vitamin can be divided into two categories：vitamins used for therapy and vitamins used for nutritional supplements. Vitamins used for therapy are selected as a deficiency；we often choose to use a single species and amount of therapeutic dose. Such as vitamin A for the treatment of night blindness；Vitamin B_1 for beriberi；vitamin B_3 for pellagra；vitamin C for scurvy；vitamin D for rickets. Vitamins used for nutritional supplements are mainly used for people with unbalanced diet. We should use more variety，small doses，frequent use or continuously，which is conducive to the absorption and utilization and can fully complement a variety of vitamins.

Vocabulary（课文词汇）

vitamin 维生素

fat-soluble 脂溶性的

deficiency 不足

alcohol 乙醇（俗称酒精）

side-effect 副作用

individual tolerance 个体耐受

dosage 剂量

supplementation 补充

nausea 恶心

diarrhoea 腹泻

vomiting 呕吐

severe 严重的

thiamine 硫胺

niacin 烟酸

pellagra 糙皮病

beriberi 脚气病

scurvy 坏血病

rickets 软骨病、佝偻病、驼背

Summary（重点小结）

1. Vitamin is a kind of trace organic substance that human and animal must

obtain from food to maintain normal physiological functions and play an important role in human growth.

2. Based on the different solubility, the vitamins can be divided into the fat-soluble vitamins and water-soluble vitamins.

3. Deficiencies of vitamins are classified as either primary or secondary.

4. Humans must consume vitamins periodically but with differing schedules, to avoid deficiency.

5. In large doses, some vitamins have documented side-effects that tend to be more severe with a larger dosage.

6. There are eight types of vitamin B: thiamin (vitamin B_1), riboflavin, niacin, pantothenic acid, vitamin B_6 (pyridoxine), biotin (vitamin B_7), folate (called folic acid when included in supplements), vitamin B_{12} (cyanocobalamin).

Quiz（课后检测）

I . **Fill in the blanks according to the information about vitamins.**

1. Vitamins _____, _____ and _____ are stored in significant amounts in the human body.

2. Deficiency of vitamin _____ is the most common cause of non-accidental blindness.

3. When side-effects emerge, recovery is often accomplished by reducing the _____ .

4. The body has a limited capacity to store most of the _____ vitamins (except B_{12} and folate, which are stored in the liver).

II . **This is the vitamin data from Chinese nutrition experts. Answer the following questions based on the information given in the figure.**

1. What can you get about vitamins from the figure?

2. How to supplement vitamin to avoid deficiency according to the actual life?

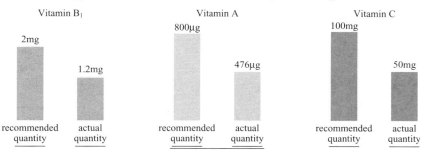

Discussion（问题讨论）

- Why can the vitamins be used to produce drugs?
- What is the application of vitamins?
- What is the difference between fat-soluble vitamins and water-soluble vitamins?
- What are the deficiencies of vitamins?
- What is the contribution of the vitamins to society?
- Why don't people get enough vitamin D?
- Why do I need vitamin?

Reading Material（延伸阅读）

Vitamin D——the healthy life come from the sun
（维生素 D——健康生活来自阳光）

Did you know that the five countries with the lowest prevalence of MS（multiple sclerosis）are Zambia，Zimbabwe，Indonesia，Cameroon，and Malawi? And the five with the highest rates are Canada，San Marino，Denmark，Sweden and Hungary. Noticed anything? It is actually true that，with just a small number of exceptions，the further away from the equator you live，the more common you'll find MS to be. But why?

Scientists think it might have something to do with the sunshine，or，more specifically，with the vitamin D that you produce through sun exposure——the sunshine vitamin.

Everyone loves a bit of sunshine，whether on holiday or at home. Maintaining a decent level of vitamin D has long been regarded as part of a healthy lifestyle. Vitamin D deficiency has been linked to a range of diseases including rickets，heart disease，cancer，depression and now MS. Of course，jetting off to the beach once a year isn't necessarily going to affect your chances of developing MS，but the research does indicate a possible link between a lack of vitamin D in early childhood and the likelihood of developing the condition. Vitamin D plays an important role in bone development，and evidence suggests it is also crucial to the immune and neuromuscular systems in the body.

Although following a healthy, balanced diet is always good for many reasons, sunlight remains the body's main source of vitamin D. A big concern among nutritionists is that our worries about over-exposure to the sun's rays have made us overly cautious in slapping on the sunscreen and preventing the body from producing the vitamin D it needs. More people are also now spending more time indoor, and the rise in obesity shows how society has become more sedentary and less active.

Part 2   Basic Technology of Separation and Purification
第二部分   分离纯化相关技术
Lesson 18   Precipitation and Dialysis
第十八课   沉淀和透析

Situational Entry（情境导入）

Biological macromolecules from a broken cell or fermented liquid contain a lot of similar or heterogeneous impurities，and it must go through a further purification. The precipitation is the common technique in the subsequent purification. We can purify target product from the mixture sample by precipitation. Due to the advantage of low cost，high yield and simple operation，the precipitation separation method is widely used in chemical industry，food industry and biochemical field. The most typical example is the extraction and separation of proteins.

Information about precipitation and dialysis（沉淀和透析的相关知识）

What is precipitation？（什么是沉淀？）

Precipitation separation is based on the principle of solubility（Fig. 18-1）.

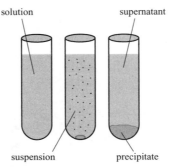

Fig. 18-1   Precipitation separation

We can choose suitable precipitant when using this technique. The precipitation is also called the solubility method. The most common precipitation separation is the salting out.

What is salting out? （什么是盐析？）

The solubility of a substance is reduced and it can be precipitated from the solution when the salt concentration of the solution exceeds a critical level. This is called salting out. Salting out is a common isolation and purification method of the proteins. The salt concentration needed for the protein to precipitate out of the solution differs from protein to protein. This process is also used to concentrate diluted solutions of proteins. Dialysis can be used to remove the salt if needed.

The mechanism of salting out （盐析的机理）

The solubility of proteins in aqueous solution is determined by two factors，hydration membrane formed between the hydrophilic groups around proteins with the water and the charge of protein. When a high concentration of neutral salt is added into the protein solution，the affinity of neutral salts to water molecules is greater than that of proteins，so the hydration membrane around protein molecules is weakened or even disappeared. At the same time，when neutral salts were added into protein solution，the surface charge of protein was neutral-

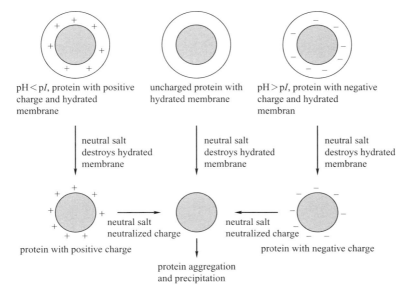

Fig. 18-2　The mechanism of salting out

ized due to the change of ionic strength, which resulted in the decrease of protein solubility and the aggregation and precipitation of protein molecules. This process is known as salting out (Fig. 18-2).

The choice of common neutral salt in salting out technique （盐析技术中中性盐的选择）

Ammonium sulfate [$(NH_4)_2SO_4$] is commonly used in the laboratory and industrial production because it has a high water solubility. The way to add ammonium sulfate to reach saturation is adding solid ammonium sulfate crystals to the sample directly. The amount of salting out ammonium sulfate required for protein precipitation is listed as below (Tab. 18-1).

Tab. 18-1　**The amount of salting out ammonium sulfate required for protein precipitation**

initial concentration of ammonium sulfate/%	percentage saturation at 0°																
	20	25	30	35	40	45	50	55	60	65	70	75	80	85	90	95	100
	solid ammonium sulfate(grams)to be added to 1 liter of solution																
0	106	134	164	194	226	258	291	326	361	398	436	476	516	559	603	650	697
5	79	108	137	166	197	229	262	296	331	368	405	444	484	526	570	615	662
10	53	81	109	139	169	200	233	266	301	337	374	412	452	493	536	581	627
15	26	54	82	111	141	172	204	237	271	306	343	381	420	460	503	547	592
20	0	27	55	83	113	143	175	207	241	276	312	349	387	427	469	512	557
25		0	27	56	84	115	146	179	211	245	280	317	355	395	436	478	522
30			0	28	56	86	117	148	181	214	249	285	323	362	402	445	488
35				0	28	57	87	118	151	184	218	254	291	329	369	410	453
40					0	29	58	89	120	153	187	222	258	296	335	376	418
45						0	29	59	90	123	156	190	226	263	302	342	383
50							0	30	60	92	125	159	194	230	265	306	348
55								0	30	61	93	127	161	197	235	273	313
60									0	31	62	95	129	164	201	239	279
65										0	31	63	97	132	168	205	244
70											0	32	65	99	134	171	209
75												0	32	66	101	137	174
80													0	33	67	103	139
85														0	34	68	105
90															0	34	70
95																0	35
100																	0

What is dialysis?（什么是透析?）

The target product often contains a high concentration of ammonium sulfate after using salting out，which can affect the subsequent purification. Therefore，neutral salt must be removed from the target product. Dialysis is a common laboratory technique utilized after salting out. It is the process of separating molecules in solution by use of semi-permeable membranes（半透膜）that permit the passage of molecules smaller than a certain size through，but prevent the passing of larger molecules. Dialysis can be used to either introduce or remove small molecules from a sample because small molecules move freely across the membrane in both directions. This makes dialysis become a technique widely used（Fig. 18-3）.

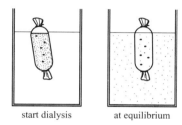

start dialysis   at equilibrium

Fig. 18-3   The dialysis of the sample after salting out

Applications（应用实例）

Precipitation reactions are often used to isolate a particular ion from the solution. The process allows selective removal of ions due to different solubilities，such as the isolation and purification of myoglobin with ammonium sulfate precipitation（Fig. 18-4）.

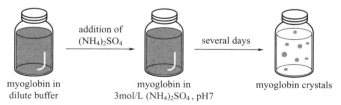

addition of $(NH_4)_2SO_4$ several days

myoglobin in   myoglobin in   myoglobin crystals
dilute buffer   3mol/L $(NH_4)_2SO_4$, pH7

Fig. 18-4   Isolation and purification of myoglobin with ammonium sulfate precipitation

Vocabulary（课文词汇）

precipitate 沉淀

salting out 盐析作用

dilute 稀释

extraction 提取

dialysis 透析

hydrophobic 疏水的

aqueous 水的，水状的

ion 离子

filtration 过滤

Summary（重点小结）

1. Biological macromolecules from a broken cell or fermented liquid contain a lot of similar or heterogeneous impurities，and it must go through further purification.

2. We can purify target product from the mixture sample by precipitation.

3. Precipitation separation is based on the principle of solubility.

4. Ammonium sulfate is the preferred neutral salt in the laboratory and industrial production.

5. The way to add ammonium sulfate to reach saturation is adding solid ammonium sulfate crystals to the sample directly.

6. Dialysis is a common laboratory technique utilized after salting out.

Quiz（课后检测）

Fill in the blanks according to the information about precipitation and dialysis.

1. _____ is the preferred neutral salt in the laboratory and industrial production.

2. Ammonium sulfate _____ is a method used to purify proteins by altering their solubility.

3. _____ is a common laboratory technique utilized after salting out.

Discussion（问题讨论）

- Why do you choose the precipitation and dialysis technique?
- What is the principle of precipitation and dialysis?
- What is the difference between precipitation and dialysis?

- What is the result of dialysis?
- Under what circumstances do we use the precipitation separation method?

Reading Material（延伸阅读）

Ammonium sulfate precipitation
（硫酸铵沉淀）

Ammonium sulfate precipitation is a method used to purify proteins by altering their solubility. It is a specific case of a more general technique known as salting out. Ammonium sulfate is commonly used, as its solubility is so high that salt solutions with high ionic strength are allowed. The solubility of proteins varies according to the ionic strength of the solution, and hence according to the salt concentration. Two distinct effects are observed: at low salt concentrations, the solubility of the protein increases with increasing salt concentration (i. e. increasing ionic strength), an effect termed salting in. As the salt concentration (ionic strength) is increased further, the solubility of the protein begins to decrease. At sufficiently high ionic strength, the protein will be almost completely precipitated from the solution (salting out).

Since proteins differ markedly in their solubilities at high ionic strength, salting out is a very useful procedure to assist in the purification of a given protein. The commonly used salt is ammonium sulfate as it is very water-soluble and forms two ions high in the Hofmeister series. Because these two ions are at the end of Hofmeister series, ammonium sulfate can also stabilize a protein structure. The ammonium sulfate solubility behavior for a protein is usually expressed as a function of the percentage of saturation.

Calculating how much ammonium sulfate to add to a solution at one concentration to achieve a desired higher concentration is tricky since the addition of ammonium sulfate significantly increases the volume of the solution. The amount to add can be determined either from published nomograms or by using an online calculator. Each protein precipitate is dissolved individually in fresh buffer and assayed for total protein content. The aim is to find the ammonium sulfate concentration which will precipitate the maximum proportion of undesired protein, whilst leaving most of the desired protein still in solution or vice versa. The precipitated protein is then removed by centrifugation and then the ammonium sulfate concentration is increased to a value that will precipitate most of the protein of interest whilst leaving the maximum amount of protein contaminants still in solution. The precipitated protein of interest is recovered by centrifugation and dissolved in fresh buffer for the next stage of purification. This technique is used to quickly remove large amounts of contaminant proteins, as the first step in many purification schemes. It is also often employed during the later stages of purification to concentrate protein from dilute solution following procedures such as gel filtration.

Lesson 19 Chromatography
第十九课 色谱分离法

🔦 Situational Entry（情境导入）

The term "chromatography" is derived from the original experiments done in Russia by the Italian-born scientist Mikhail Tsvet for separating yellow and green plant pigment in 1903-1906 (Fig. 19-1，and see colored picture). Chromatography is an analytical technique commonly used for separating a mixture of chemical substances into its individual components，so that the individual components can be thoroughly analyzed. The components to be separated are distributed between two phases，a stationary phase bed and a mobile phase that percolates through the stationary bed.

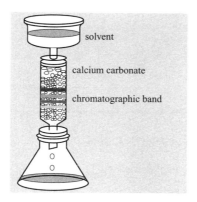

Fig. 19-1   The experiment of the separating yellow and green plant pigment
stationary phase：calcium carbonate；mobile phase：solvent

Information about chromatography（色谱分离法的相关知识）

What is chromatography?（什么是色谱分离法?）

Chromatography is the collective term for a set of laboratory techniques for the separation of mixtures. The technique is based on the difference of physical and chemical properties of different substances. All the chromatographic systems consist of two phases, stationary phase and mobile phase.

Classification of chromatographic techniques（色谱分离技术的分类）

All chromatographic techniques are used for the separation of a mixture that contains a few components, such as the separation of proteins. The sample is dissolved in the mobile phase. When it flows through the stationary phase, different components in the sample are separated because of different distribution ratios between stationary and mobile phases. And after some time, they will be distributed in spaces over the stationary phase and subsequently elute out of the stationary phase as single components. Several types of chromatography and their stationary and mobile phases are listed below (Tab. 19-1).

Tab. 19-1   Types of chromatography

mobile phase	stationary phase	technique
liquid	liquid	partition chromatography
gas	liquid	gas-liquid chromatography
gas	solid	gas-solid chromatography
liquid	ion exchange resin	ion exchange chromatography
liquid	molecular sieves	ion exclusion/gel permeation
liquid	thin layer of silica/alumina	thin layer chromatography
liquid	paper	paper chromatography

Chromatography terms（色谱分离法术语）

Analyte: proteins or saccharides to be separated.

Chromatogram: the visual output of the time distribution of the detected signals of the separated components. Different peaks or patterns on the chromatogram correspond to different components of the separated mixture.

Stationary phase: the substance fixed in place for the chromatography procedure and can separate and preserve the sample. The selection of stationary phase plays an important and sometimes decisive role in the separation of samples.

Mobile phase: carries the sample being separated/analyzed and moves through the stationary phase where the sample interacts with and is separated.

Column chromatography: a technique for separation of biomolecules. The stationary phase is packed into a tube or concentrated on or along the inside tube wall, mobile phase mixed with the samples flows through the stationary bed (Fig. 19-2).

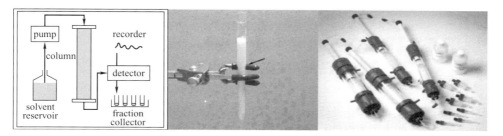

Fig. 19-2   Column chromatography

Gel filtration chromatography（凝胶过滤色谱）

What is gel filtration chromatography?（什么是凝胶过滤色谱？）

Gel column chromatography is mainly used to separate molecules of different sizes. The solution with the sample containing different sizes of molecules is poured into a column, which is packed with porous beads made of a cross-linked polymeric material (such as dextran or agarose). Molecules larger than the pores can't enter the bead, which is excluded, and move quickly through the column. Molecules smaller than the pores can enter the bead, which is retarded, and medium-size molecules partially enter the bead. As a result, molecules of different sizes are separated (Fig. 19-3, and see colored picture).

The process of gel filtration chromatography（凝胶过滤色谱的过程）

The process of gel filtration chromatography is listed below.

1. Choosing suitable gel medium, then pack spherical particles of gel filtration medium into a column.

2. The sample is applied to the column. Sample volume should not exceed 1-5% of column bed volume.

3. Add buffer. Buffer and sample move through the column. Molecules diffuse in and out of the pores of the matrix.

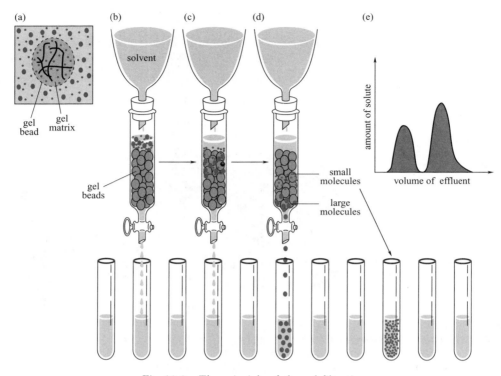

Fig. 19-3　The principle of the gel filtration

4. As buffer passes through the column，molecules that do not enter the matrix are eluted. Molecules with partial access to the pores of the matrix elute from the column in the order of decreasing size.

5. In general，liquid chromatography systems are equipped with partial collectors to collect samples. It is commonly used to collect separated molecules according to the prescribed time or volume of eluent. Separated molecules can also be collected according to the elution peak detected by the detector.

Applications（应用实例）

Gel chromatography can be used for desalting after salting out. The protein mixed with the salt solution flows through gel column，salt and protein with small molecule weight enter into the pores of the gel particles and move downward slowly，while protein with large molecular weight cannot enter the pores of the gel particles，and has a faster flowing rate through gel column，which makes the protein and salt separate. Such as using Sephadex G-25 desalting proteins in

Fig. 19-4. The first peak is the protein, the second peak is the salt removed from the protein.

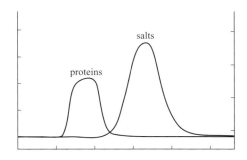

Fig. 19-4   Sephadex G-25 desalting from the proteins

Ion exchange chromatography（IEX）（离子交换色谱）

What is ion exchange chromatography?（什么是离子交换色谱？）

Ion-exchange chromatography（or ion chromatography）is one of the most widely used methods for purification of biological macromolecules. The sample containing different components is separated by ion exchanger as stationary phase, and the difference of binding force formed by reversible exchange of components in mobile phase and equilibrium ions on exchanger.

Principles of ion exchange chromatography（离子交换色谱的原理）

Biomolecules have different affinity with ion exchangers because of their different anions, cations and charges. When the ionic strength and pH value of solution are changed, different biomolecules can be separated from the column in turn. Proteins, which are built up of many different amino acids containing weak acidic and basic groups, their net surface charge changes with pH in a manner that is dictated by a protein's isoelectric point（pI）(Fig. 19-5).

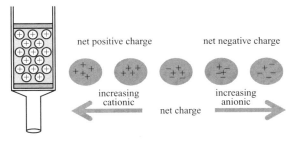

Fig. 19-5   The principle of the ion exchange chromatography

Let's take the separation of proteins as an example. When proteins containing different components flow through the ion columns, the separation of target proteins can be effectively achieved by choosing the appropriate acidity, basicity and ionic strength of the equilibrium buffer. The component in the proteins with the lowest net charge at the selected pH will be the first ones eluted from the column (small orange ball in Fig. 19-6, and see colored picture). Similarly, the component in proteins with the highest charge at a certain pH will be most strongly retained and will be eluted last (small blue ball in Fig. 19-6, and see colored picture). The net surface charges of proteins are different, which results in the different binding strength. The components in the proteins can be separated and eluted one by one by gradually increasing salt concentration of the buffer, i. e. ionic strength. With the increase of ionic strength, the salt ions (typically Na^+ or Cl^-) compete with the bound components for charges on the surface of the medium, resulting in the gradual elution of the components (Fig. 19-6).

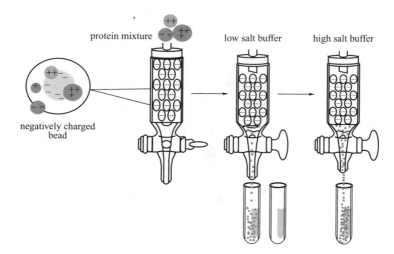

Fig. 19-6　The elution due to the increases of ionic strength

Ion exchanger (离子交换剂)

Ion exchangers are insoluble macromolecule substances containing several ionic groups, which are prepared by adding several dissociable groups (active groups) into insoluble macromolecule substances (parent). The materials of the matrix can be resin, cellulose, acrylamide gel, Sephadex. They are usually porous to give a high internal surface area. The medium is packed into a column to form a packed bed. The bed is then equilibrated with a buffer, which fills the pores of the matrix and the space between the particles. According to the properties of active groups, ionic agents can be divided into cation exchangers and anion exchangers. A positively charged medium is also named anion exchanger; a negatively charged medium is also called cation exchanger. The ion exchanger can be divided into ion exchange resin, ion exchange cellulose and ion exchange gel according to the difference of the matrix.

Ion exchange resin（离子交换树脂）

Ion exchange resin is the typical ion exchanger. The main properties and types of resins are determined by the types of chemical active groups in resins. It can be divided into cation resins and anion resins, which can exchange cations and anions in solution respectively. Cation exchanger can be divided into strong acidity and weak acidity. Anion exchanger can be divided into strong alkalinity and weak alkalinity. There are also amphoteric exchangers that are able to exchange both cations and anions simultaneously. At a pH above its isoelectric point, a protein will bind to a positively charged medium or anion exchanger. At a pH below its pI, a protein will bind to a negatively charged medium or cation exchanger (Fig. 19-7).

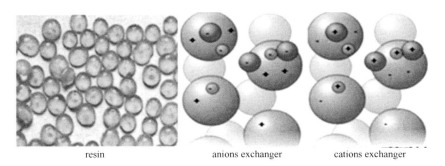

resin   anions exchanger   cations exchanger

Fig. 19-7   The anion exchanger and cation exchanger

Ion exchange chromatography workflow（离子交换色谱的工作流程）

All ion exchange chromatography relies on electrostatic interactions between the resin functional groups and proteins of interest. Its workflow is listed below (Fig. 19-8).

Step 1: The eluent is loaded onto the column, making the resin surface and the eluent anion saturated.

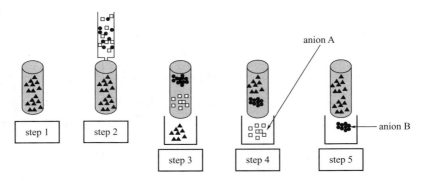

Fig. 19-8   The process of the ion exchange chromatography

Step 2：Here we use a sample containing two anions as an example. A sample containing anion A and anion B is injected into the column.

Step 3：After adding the sample，more eluent is added. The eluent carried the sample through the column. Anion A and B were attached to the column surface in different ways.

Step 4：As the eluent continues to be added，the anion A moves through the column in a band and ultimately is eluted first.

Step 5：With the increase of eluent concentration，the binding force between anion and resin decreases，the eluent displaces anion B，and anion B is eluted off the column.

Applications（应用实例）

Ion-exchange chromatography can be applied to almost all kinds of charged molecule including large proteins，small nucleotides and amino acids.

The deionized water is widely used in laboratories. Ion-exchange chromatography is used in preparation of deionized water（Fig. 19-9）. A series of cation exchange columns and anion exchange columns are used. The cation exchange resins are used to remove various cations，while anion exchange resin is used to remove various anions.

Affinity chromatography（亲和色谱）

What is affinity chromatography?（什么是亲和色谱？）

Affinity chromatography is a method for the separation and specific analysis of sample components，which based on a highly specific interaction such as that

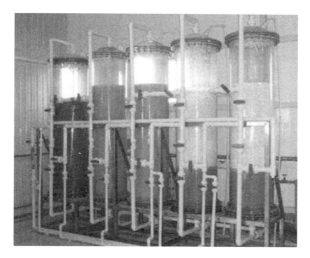

Fig. 19-9 The preparation of deionized water by ion exchange chromatography

between an immobilized ligand and its binding partner. It is very effective for separating proteins, which usually requires only one step to obtain a high purity protein of interest. It has the advantages of high selectivity, high recovery efficiency, high purity.

Biomolecules with typical biological affinity are enzyme and substrate, inhibitor and cofactor, antibody and antigen, virus and cell lectin, polysaccharide and glycoprotein, cell surface and receptor, poly-His-tag fused proteins, native proteins with histidine, hormone, and receptor (Fig. 19-10).

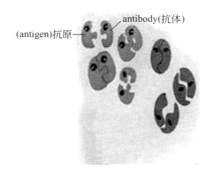

Fig. 19-10 The process of using affinity chromatography

Principle of affinity chromatography（亲和色谱的原理）

Affinity chromatography is based on reversible binding between biological molecules and their ligands, just like a lock to a key. The reversible binding mainly depends on the recognition of the spatial structure of biopolymers and their ligands.

We illustrate the principle of affinity chromatography using the separation of proteins as an example below (Fig. 19-11, and see colored picture).

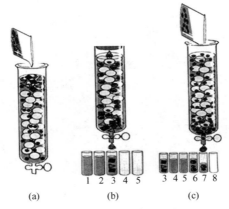

(a)   (b)   (c)

Fig. 19-11   Principle of ion affinity chromatography

The ligand with specific affinity for the protein of interest is immobilized on the insoluble carrier and packed into the column. When the protein mixture is added to the column [Fig. 19-11(a)], only the protein of interest in the mixture is adsorbed and can react with the ligand to form a complex. The unwanted proteins [Fig. 19-11(b), (c)-3] that do not coordinate are washed away through the column. At this time, only the target protein remains in the column, and then a high concentration eluent of the interested protein ligand was added [Fig. 19-11 (c)]. Because the ligand concentration in the eluent is higher than that in the column, the interested protein could be separated by combining the ligand in the eluent and dissociating the fixed ligand [Fig. 19-11(c)-6,7]. As a result, purifications that would otherwise be time-consuming and complicated or even impossible can often be easily achieved with affinity chromatography.

Affinity chromatography medium（亲和色谱介质）

Affinity chromatography medium is obtained by chemical bonding of affinity ligands to the chromatography medium. The ideal medium of affinity chromatography should meet the following requirement. (1) Insoluble in water, highly hydrophilic. (2) Inertia, less non-specific adsorption. (3) Chemical groups with a considerable amount of activation. (4) Stable physical and chemical properties. (5) Good mechanical properties. (6) Good permeability, porous network structure. (7) Resistant to microorganisms and alcohols.

The process of using affinity chromatography （亲和色谱操作过程） (Fig. 19-12)

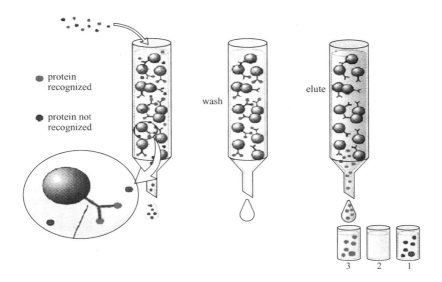

Fig. 19-12   The process of affinity chromatography

Step 1：Prepare the solid-phase with special affinity molecule and place in the column.

Step 2：Equilibrate the medium and sample to binding conditions.

Step 3：Apply the sample and wash out contaminants. When the protein mixture to be separated passes through the column，the affinity protein with the adsorbent would be adsorbed and retained in the column. Those proteins without affinity flow out directly because they are not adsorbed，so they are separated.

Step 4：Desorb and elute the target. The proteins that are bound can be eluted by changing the binding conditions using the appropriate eluent.

Step 5：Re-equilibrate the medium to binding conditions.

Applications（应用实例）

The diversity of antibody-antigen interactions has created many uses for antibodies and antibody fragments. The potential exists to create an infinite number of combinations between immunoglobulins and immunoglobulin fragments with tags and other selected proteins.

Vocabulary（课文词汇）

chromatography 色谱

gel filtration 凝胶过滤

ion exchange 离子交换

affinity chromatography 亲和色谱

analyte 被分析物

stationary phase 固定相

mobile phase 流动相

matrix 基质

spherical 球形的

capacity 容量

acrylamide 丙烯酰胺

Sephadex 葡聚糖

cation 阳离子

anion 阴离子

equilibration buffer 平衡缓冲液

elute 洗脱

glycoprotein 甘氨酸

Summary（重点小结）

1. Gel filtration is the simplest and mildest one of all the chromatography techniques and separates molecules on the basis of differences in size.

2. Ion-exchange chromatography（or ion chromatography）is a process that allows the separation of ions and polar molecules based on their affinity to the ion exchanger.

3. Affinity chromatography is a method of separating biochemical mixtures based on a highly specific interaction.

4. Ion exchangers are either cation exchangers that exchange positively charged ions（cations）or anion exchangers that exchange negatively charged ions（anions）.

Quiz（课后检测）

Ⅰ. **Fill in the blanks according to the information about chromatography.**

1. The proteins with the _____ net charge at the selected pH will be the first ones eluted from the column as ionic strength increases.

2. Affinity binding is the _____ and _____ analogy.

3. Ion exchange _____ is the typical ion exchanger.

Ⅱ. **Analyze the following pictures according to the knowledge about the affinity chromatography.**

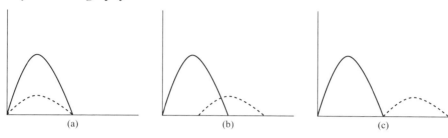

(a)　　　　　　　　　(b)　　　　　　　　　(c)

Discussion（问题讨论）

- Why do you choose the chromatography technique?
- What is the principle of chromatography?
- What is the difference between gel chromatography and affinity chromatography?
- What is the result of chromatography?

Reading Material（延伸阅读）

Isolation of caffeine from tea
（从茶叶中分离咖啡因）

Caffeine often needs to be isolated from tea leaves. The major problem of the isolation is that caffeine does not occur alone in tea leaves，but is accompanied by other natural substances from which it must be separated.

The major component of tea leaves is cellulose，which is the major structural material of all plant cells. Cellulose is a polymer of glucose. Since cellulose is virtually insoluble in water，it presents no problems in the isolation procedure. Caffeine，on the other hand，is water soluble and is one of the major substances extracted from the solution called "tea". It comprises as much as 5% by weight of the leaf material in tea plants. Tannins also dissolve in the hot water used to extract tea leaves.

The term tannin does not refer to a single homogeneous compound，or even to substances which have similar chemical structure. It refers to a class of compounds that have certain properties in common. Tannins are phenolic compounds having molecular weights between 500 and 3000. They are widely used to "tan" leather. They precipitate alkaloids and proteins from aqueous solutions. Tannins are usually divided into two classes: those can be hydrolyzed and those cannot. Tannins of the first type found in tea generally yield glucose and gallic acid when they are hydrolyzed. These tannins are esters of gallic acid and glucose. They represent structures in which some of the hydroxyl groups in glucose have been esterified by diallyl groups. The non-hydrolyzable tannins found in tea are condensation polymers of catechin. These polymers are not uniform in structure, but catechin molecules are usually linked together at ring positions 4 and 8. When tannins are extracted into hot water, the hydrolyzable ones are partially hydrolyzed, meaning that free gallic acid is also found in tea. The tannins, by virtue of their phenolic groups, and gallic acid by virtue of its carboxyl groups, are both acidic. If calcium carbonate, a base, is added to tea water, the calcium salts of these acids are formed. Caffeine can be extracted from the basic tea solution with chloroform, but the calcium salts of gallic acid and the tannins are not chloroform soluble and remain behind in the aqueous solution.

The brown color of a tea solution is due to flavonoid pigments and chlorophylls, as well as their respective oxidation products. Although chlorophylls are somewhat chloroform soluble, most of the other substances in tea are not. Thus, the chloroform extraction of the basic tea solution removes the nearly pure caffeine. The chloroform can be easily removed by distillation (at 61℃) to leave the crude caffeine. The caffeine may be purified by recrystallization or by sublimation.

Appendix
附　录

Vocabulary on Pharmaceutical English
(常用药学专业相关词汇)

1. Adj：药用辅料（pharmaceutic adjuvant）

稀释剂（diluent agent）

黏合剂（binder）

崩解剂（disintegrating agent）

润滑剂（lubricant）

基质（base）

芳香剂（flavoring agent）

甜味剂（sweetening agent）

着色剂（coloring agent）

防腐剂（preservative or antiseptics）

抗氧化剂（antioxidant）

包衣剂（coating material）

成膜材料（film-forming material）

溶剂（solvent）

增溶剂（solubilizer）

润湿剂（wetting agent or moistening agent）

吸附剂（absorbent）

助滤剂（filtering aid）

乳化剂（emulsifying agent）

表面活性剂（surfactant）

助悬剂（suspending agent）

增稠剂（viscosity increasing agent）

增塑剂（plasticizer）

螯合剂（chelating agent）

透皮促进剂（transdermal enhancer）

气雾抛射剂（aerosol propellant）

起泡剂（foaming agent）

酸碱调节剂（acidifying or alkalizing agent）

缓冲剂（buffering agent）

2. Aer：气雾剂（aerosol）

吸入气雾剂（inhalation aerosol）

吸入粉雾剂（powder for inhalation）

非吸入气雾剂（non-inhalation aerosol）

外用气雾剂（topical aerosol，skin aerosol）

喷雾剂（spray）

药用泡沫剂（medicated foam，cutaneous foam）

鼻腔用喷雾剂（nasal spray）

3. Cap：胶囊剂（capsule）

硬胶囊剂（hard capsule）

软胶囊剂（soft capsule）

肠溶胶囊剂（enteric-coated capsule，enteric-microencapsulated capsule，gastro-resistant capsule，delayed-release capsule）

缓释胶囊剂（sustained-release capsule，extended-release capsule）

控释胶囊剂（controlled-release capsule，modified-release capsule）

直肠用胶囊（rectal capsule）

4. EarD：滴耳剂（ear drop）

溶液型滴耳液（otic solution）

混悬型滴耳液（otic suspension）

洗耳剂（ear wash）

5. EyeD：滴眼剂（eye drop）

溶液型滴眼剂（ophthalmic solution）

混悬型滴眼剂（ophthalmic suspension）

眼内注射溶液（intraocular solution）

眼用洗剂（eye lotion）

6. EyeO：眼膏剂（eye ointment，ophthalmic ointment）

眼用乳膏（ophthalmic cream）

眼用凝胶（ophthalmic gel）

7. Gel：凝胶剂（gel）

混悬凝胶剂（otic gel）

局部用凝胶剂（topical gel）

胶浆剂（mucilage，jelly）

火棉胶剂（collodion）

8. Gran：颗粒剂（granule）

细粒剂（fine granules，micro-granule）

可溶颗粒剂（soluble granule）

混悬颗粒剂（suspension granule）

泡腾颗粒剂（effervescent granule）

肠溶颗粒剂（gastro-resistant granule）

缓释颗粒剂（sustained-release granule）

控释颗粒剂（controlled-release granule）

9. Inj：注射剂（injection）

乳状液（injectable emulsion）

混悬液（injectable suspension）

静脉滴注用输液（intravenous infusion）

注射用灭菌粉末（powder for injection）

注射用浓溶液（concentrated solution for injection）

植入剂（implant，insert）

10. Lin：搽剂（liniment）

11. Lot：洗剂（lotion）

12. NasD：滴鼻剂（nasal drop）

鼻腔用溶液（intra-nasal solution）

鼻腔用混悬液（intra-nasal suspension）

洗鼻液（nasal wash）

鼻用胶浆（nasal jelly）

13. Oint：软膏剂（ointment）

乳膏剂（cream）

糊剂（paste）

阴道霜剂（vaginal cream）

14. OraL：口服制剂

口服液体制剂（oral liquid）

口服溶液剂（oral solution）

口服混悬剂（oral suspension）

口服乳剂 （oral emulsion）

口服滴剂 （oral drop）

口服干混悬剂 （for oral suspension）

合剂 （mixture）

酏剂 （elixir）

乳浆剂 （magma）

15. Pat：贴剂 （patch）

透皮贴剂 （transdermal patch）

16. Pel：膜剂 （pellicle）

口服膜剂 （oral pellicle）

黏膜外用药膜 （film）

牙周条 （strip）

17. Pil：丸剂 （pill）

滴丸 （dripping pill）

糖丸 （sugared pill）

耳丸 （ear pellet，otic pellet）

眼丸 （eye pellet，ophthalmic pellet，ocular system）

小丸 （pellet）

缓释小丸 （sustained-release pellet）

18. Powd：散剂 （powder）

内服散剂 （oral powder）

局部用散剂 （topical powder）

撒布剂 （dusting powder）

口服泡腾散剂 （effervescent oral powder）

19. Sol：溶液剂 （solution）

局部用溶液 （topical solution）

灌肠剂 （enema）

直肠用溶液 （rectal solution）

灌洗液 （irrigation solution）

透析液 （dialysis solution）

含漱液 （gargle，oral rinse，mouthwash）

吸入溶液剂 （inhalation solution）

雾化用溶液 （solution for atomization）

20. Sup：栓剂（suppository）

直肠栓（rectal suppository）

阴道栓剂（vaginal suppository，pessary）

21. Syr：糖浆剂（syrup）

干糖浆（dry syrup）

舐剂（或称润喉止咳糖浆 linctus）

22. Tab：片剂（tablet）

普通片（uncoated tablet）

包衣片（coated tablet，film-coated table，sugar-coated tablet）

口含片（buccal tablet，troches）

舌下片（sublingual tablet）

咀嚼片（chewable tablet）

分散片（dispersible tablet）

泡腾片（effervescent tablet）

阴道片（vaginal tablet）

阴道泡腾片（vaginal effervescent tablet）

速释片（rapid-release tablet）

缓释片（sustained-release tablet、extended-release tablet or prolonged-release tablet）

控释片（controlled-release tablet、accelerated-release tablet or pulsatile-release tablet）

肠溶片（enteric-coated tablet or gastro-resistant tablet or delayed-release tablet）

口分散片（orodispersible tablet）

纸型片（chart tablet）

口腔粘贴片（muco-adhesive tablet）

溶液片（soluble tablet）

外用片（tablets for external use 或 topical solutions tablet）

模制片（molded tablet）

锭剂（lozenge 或 pastille）

23. Tin：酊剂（tincture）

醑剂（spirit）

24. 其他剂型

敷贴（application）

芳香水剂（aromatic water）

胶接剂（cement）

浸蘸用（for dip）

流浸膏（fluid extract）

胶姆剂（gums）

柠檬水剂（lemonade）

脂质体（liposome）

皮肤敷贴用液体制剂（liquid for cutaneous application）

药用咀嚼胶姆剂（medicated chewing gum）

药用泡沫剂（medicated foam）

微球（microsphere）

指甲液或涂剂（nail solution or nail lacquer）

眼用植入剂（ophthalmic insert）

醋蜜剂（oxymel）

涂抹（paint）

Reference
（参考文献）

[1] Dore A J, Mousavi-Baygi M, Smith R I, Hall J, Fowler D and Choularton T W, 2006. A model of annual orographic precipitation and acid deposition and its application to Snowdonia. Atmosphere Environment, 2006, 40 (18): 3316-3326.

[2] Anonymous commentator. 1998. An important reform on the mechanism of drug evaluation. China Pharmaceutical News.

[3] Bailon Pascal, Ehrlich George K. Fung Wen-Jian, Berthold Wolfgang. 2000. An Overview of Affinity Chromatography. Humana Press.

[4] Bender N Human. 2010. Biology and Health. Quarterly Review of Biology.

[5] Yuan B, Wu H. 1998. Present situation, problems and countermeasures of the new drug research and development in China. Chinese Journal of New Drugs.

[6] Cavalier-Smith T. 1998. A revised six-kingdom system of life. Biol Rev Camb Philos Soc, 1998, 73 (3): 203-206.

[7] Qi M. 1988. The Development of Pharmacy In Contemporary China. Beijing: China Social Sciences Press.

[8] Ettre L S. 1993. Nomenclature for chromatography IUPAC Recommendations. Pure and Applied Chemistry.

[9] Emmanouil N Anagnostou. 2004. A convective/stratiform precipitation classification algorithm for volume scanning weather radar observations. Meteorological Applications (Cambridge University Press).

[10] Dong H, et al. 1999. Drug policy in China: pharmaceutical distribution in rural area. Social Science & Medicine.

[11] Kaczmarek, Jakubowska N, et al. 2016. The microorganisms of cryoconite holes (algae, Archaea, bacteria, cyanobacteria, fungi, and Protista): a review. Polar Record.

[12] Kastoris A C, Rafailidis P I, Vouloumanou E K, et al. 2010. Synergy of fosfomycin with other antibiotics for Gram-positive and Gram-negative bacteria. European Journal of Clinical Pharmacology.

[13] Wang K. 1994. Historical materials: medical chapter 1949-1990. Beijing Science and Technology Press.

[14] Moran M. 2002. Understanding the regulatory state. British Journal of Political Science.

[15] Migliori G B, Besozzi G, Girardi E, et al. 2007. Clinical and operational value of the extensively drug-resistant tuberculosis definition. European Respiratory Journal.

[16] Mucciolo L F. 1975. Scientific Reduction and the Mind-Body Problem. Canadian journal of philosophy.

[17] Miller S A, Dykes D D, Polesky H F. 1988. A simple salting out procedure for extracting DNA from human nucleated cells. Nucleic acids research.

[18] Nair P C, Miners J O. 2014. Molecular dynamics simulations: from structure function relationships to drug discovery. In Silico Pharmacology.

[19] Simoni R D, Hill R L, Vaughan M. The Structure and Function of Hemoglobin: Gilbert Smithson

Adair and the Adair Equations [J]. Journal of Biological Chemistry, 2002, 277 (31): e20.

[20] Uhlén M. 2008. Affinity as a tool in life science. Biotechniques.

[21] Still W C, Kahn M, Mitra A. 1978. Rapid chromatographic technique for preparative separations with moderate resolution. J Org Chem.

[22] Van Holde K E. 1998. Analytical ultracentrifugation from 1924 to the present: A remarkable history. Chemtracts-Biochemistry and Molecular Biology.

[23] Vinod J, Chenthilnathan A, Vijayakumar S . 2013. Formulation and Evaluation of Modified Release Matrix Tablets of Trimetazidine Dihydrochloride. International Journal for Pharmaceutical Research Scholars.

[24] Zhang X. 2003. Discipline of Drug Policy. Beijing: Science Press.

[25] Weibel E R. The oxygen pathway: how well-built is the respiratory system? Schweizerische Medizinische Wochenschrift, 1994, 124 (7): 282.

[26] Elseviers M, Wettermark B, Almarsdóttir, Anna Birna, et al. Drug Utilization Research (Methods and Applications) Introduction to drug utilization research. John Wiley & Sons, Ltd, 2016.

[27] Katsura, Toshiya. Journal of Pharmaceutical Health Care and Sciences. Journal of Pharmaceutical Health Care and Sciences, 2015, 1 (1): 1.

[28] Zhi L, Lan C, Ying H, et al. Advances in research on immune organs and immunocytes of nonhuman primates. Chinese Journal of Pharmacology and Toxicology, 2013.

[29] Li H, Sun H. The Historical Evolution Of China's Drug Regulatory System. Value in Health, 2014, 17 (3): A30-A31.

[30] Zimm B H, Levene S D. 1992. Problems and prospects in the theory of gel electrophoresis of DNA. Quarterly Reviews of Biophysics.